Living Yoga Wisdom

Philosophical Exercises for Personal Practice

Living Yoga Wisdom

Philosophical Exercises for Personal Practice

Eckard Wolz-Gottwald

Translation by Ilka Schröder

MANTRA
BOOKS

Winchester, UK
Washington, USA

First published by Mantra Books, 2015
Mantra Books is an imprint of John Hunt Publishing Ltd., Laurel House, Station Approach,
Alresford, Hants, SO24 9JH, UK
office1@jhpbooks.net
www.johnhuntpublishing.com
www.mantra-books.net

For distributor details and how to order please visit the 'Ordering' section on our website.

The original edition of *Living Yoga Wisdom - Philosophical Exercises for Personal Practice* was
first published in 2009 under the title *Yoga-Weisheit leben. Philosophische Übungen für die
Praxis* by Via Nova, Petersberg/Germany (2nd edition 2014)

Grateful acknowledgment is made to Maria Richardson for proofreading the first edition in the
English language.

ISBN: 978 1 78279 639 8
Library of Congress Control Number: 2014956729

A CIP catalogue record for this book is available from the British Library.

Design: Stuart Davies

Printed and bound by CPI Group (UK) Ltd, Croydon, CR0 4YY, UK

We operate a distinctive and ethical publishing philosophy in all
areas of our business, from our global network of authors to
production and worldwide distribution.

CONTENTS

Introduction

From theory to philosophy as a practice

Living Yoga Wisdom is a practice book of yoga philosophy. The book conveys background knowledge and the theoretic basics of yoga. It explains how yoga works and what is meant by transformation, awakening and enlightenment. It also reveals the theory of practice. In this book the big topics of yoga are interpreted in a manner that are relevant for life, starting with the question of reincarnation, the philosophy of OM and the search for divine and self-experiences.

As crucial as these theories are they, however, only form the surface of what yoga really is. Consequently, yoga philosophy means a lot more. Theories *on* yoga can only constitute an outer layer, but they cannot be the actual fruit of yoga philosophy. The theories are the starting point from where to immerse into the depths of one's own experiences. This way yoga philosophy turns into a path of practice. Every chapter in this book provides concrete practical exercises for reflection, through which yoga philosophy will not only become comprehensible, but can be applied practically and becomes experiential. Thus, the teachings of yoga philosophy transform from theories on yoga into experiences of yoga philosophy. Yoga philosophy turns into a practice of consciousness training.

In practice traditionally yoga philosophy is considered the "highest means of catharsis", but what does catharsis actually mean in this context? Catharsis means cleansing, but it is not about outer cleansing like using soap to clean your hands. The dirt that is referred to in this context are tensions in body and mind, unconsciousness, urges and addictions. Yoga philosophy becomes a practice of inner catharsis, if we can manage to go beyond the theoretical learning of the principles of the yogic path and apply the philosophy for ourselves. If we can manage to perceive ourselves in our own unconsciousness, work with it and begin to walk the path of consciousness training, then yoga is not only about understanding how it can transform people, but it is about our own initial experiences of transformation. Yoga philosophy as practice means contemplating the principles of being human. It shows the path of experiencing the depth of our very own existence.

In the beginning, aids are given in order to understand the world theoretically. Then, it is important to develop consciousness of our own deep involvement within the cosmos. Initially, it is about the theoretical principles of yogic ethics, which mean rules and commandments of good conduct. As a practice yoga philosophy trains our consciousness for good conduct from the depth of our very own existence. Going beyond the accumulation of theoretical knowledge, now wisdom can grow – wisdom of body, mind and soul. Even if yoga philosophy aims to teach in the beginning, its very objective is to awaken humanity. The wisdom that is referred to is one that has not been uttered through spoken language yet. The words of yoga philosophy point towards a hidden treasure within us, which will be discovered once we begin to live yoga.

Yoga philosophy as an ascent up a mountain

We can picture practicing yoga philosophy as the preparation, the aids and perhaps also provisions for an ascent up a mountain. Understanding the theories of yoga asks for a lot of effort and comprehensive studies. Yoga theories impress through their complexities and conciseness. Theoretical knowledge on yoga can provide a foothold and stability. The more knowledge we accumulate the more stable grounds we can gain underneath our feet.

However, all contemplation and all theories on yoga are only like the preliminary circling around a mountain, which we are actually supposed to climb. Complicated theories take complicated routes. Easy theories make it somewhat easier. Yet, one still remains at the bottom in the foothills of the mountain. Some yoga theorists do not even know that there is something like a mountain. Others believe they have already climbed up high and interpret their moves as though they are about to reach the summit. Despite all movement that they cause, the theories themselves do not lead to an ascent.

Yoga philosophy in its deeper sense means the risk of ascending up a mountain. But when does the ascent finally take place? Ascending means the application of the knowledge of yoga to ourselves and walking the path of transformation. Yoga philosophy becomes a practice of thinking once, not only insight on yoga, but also insight on ourselves grows. Climbing the mountain of yoga means to transform oneself. And we transform once tensions, unconsciousness and urges begin to be released and thus clarity of our true Self starts to emerge. At the same time, ascending to yoga philosophy can be a difficult climb, but this does not need to be the case. Some are being inspired by simple stories of yoga philosophy. Others prefer thought-provoking challenges and are more drawn to the abstract, harder to understand language of the *Yoga Sutras*. The only importance is to be open for change when immersing oneself in yoga philosophy, so that consciousness and insight can grow. Only if yoga philosophy turns into a practice in this manner, one can rightfully speak of yoga philosophy as "the highest means of catharsis".

Unfolding the full potential of yoga

Yoga does not only mean exercising the body. The physical exercise of yoga nowadays is the most widespread form of yoga. Like physical exercises exercise the body, breathing exercises exercise the breath. Yoga meditation works with mental objects, yoga philosophy works with thought. Yoga philosophy represents itself as one single limb in a large network of the various pathways of yoga. Through this network of the various paths of yoga we are provided with a broad spectrum of opportunities that are to be utilized. The various ways of practice can reciprocate and support each other in order to unfold their full potential. The physical and breathing exercises will ground the yogic philosopher, and vice versa the practice of yoga philosophy can intensify our physical practice. In the reciprocal enrichment and support of the various forms of practice lies a great chance, which shows us the variety of the yogic ways. Clarity increases on the actual purpose of the physical practice. We can conclude better whether we are on the right path with our practice or whether we have been entering a blind alley; whether the chosen practice suits us or whether another form of practice should be chosen. In this way, yoga philosophy helps us to experience the original sense of our own practice, and to acknowledge what yoga is and what it wants. The objective is not only to deepen our knowledge on yoga, but more so to expand the consciousness of our own practice. It is about a better understanding of what we are actually doing when we are practicing yoga. The insights of yoga philosophy support our practice with body, breath and also with meditation.

However, the full potential of yoga will only unfold if it becomes clear that yoga practice is not limited to practice times only such as once a week in a course, or perhaps even daily on your own mat. Then yoga philosophy fosters not only a more conscious practice but also a more conscious life. The purpose of yoga philosophy is only achieved once it becomes clear that yoga is a way of life, which has been expressed since ancient times in the Sanskrit term *sadhana*. Yoga as *sadhana* means that the entire life turns into a field of practice – a practice of a comprehensive consciousness for a genuine and original life from the inner center. Experiencing yoga philosophy means change, transformation and growth in order to become more aware of what really matters in life.

From acrobatic thinking to transformation and growth

But what exactly is the mastery of yoga? Are those easy physical exercises, where the arms are lifted and lowered in a conscious manner, worth less than those difficult poses, which require high flexibility and fitness? Some consider a headstand or the lotus seat the ideal of a yoga practice, but they confuse yoga with physical acrobatics in this way. An acrobat may impress other people, especially when exposing his yoga arts, but that does not necessarily mean that he is a better yogi or a better yogini.

The physical exercises of yoga allow us to live from the center, when the practice starts to transform the practitioner, when tightness and tensions begin to loosen, when ease and concentration emerge, when consciousness of body and mind increases. Some need the challenge, the body workout including a shower after their practice. For yoga, however, it is important that growth and transformation can happen. Yoga works if the exercises enable a process of growth – growth in liveliness and consciousness from the depth of the inner center.

What applies to physical exercise is also true for yoga philosophy. Many believe yoga philosophy must be hard and complicated, abstract and full of Sanskrit terms. The physical acrobat as well as the thinking acrobat may impress people through their extraordinary abilities, but like physical acrobatics are not genuine yoga, so yoga philosophy as acrobatic thinking only touches a very outer layer of yoga and not the inner life. The inner sense of yoga philosophy refers to a way of thinking that changes the practitioner. Yoga philosophy in its original sense becomes a way of experience. Yoga philosophy means to go on an expedition for the hidden treasure of yoga, which rests deep inside of us. The traditions of yoga philosophy, of which some are thousands of years old, can help us to experience this treasure today.

How to practice yoga philosophy?

In this practice book you will find both easy and also rather demanding texts. Demonstrative and memorable images are being used. You will also find that terms from Sanskrit are continuously being introduced. It is not necessary, however, to work through one chapter after another, because each topic constitutes an independent unit respectively. Please feel free to choose your way into this book according to your very own interests. If knowledge on the historical backgrounds of yoga is important to you, you may want to start with the first part of this book. If essentially you want to understand better what is happening to you on the yogic path, you may want to start with the second part of this book, the philosophy of the yogic pathway. However, it is indeed also possible to begin with philosophy as a practice in the third part of this book or with one of the big topics of yoga philosophy in the fourth part.

Each chapter is coupled with exercises that will help to not only make yoga philosophy comprehensible but also experiential. Here the rule of thumb is: less is more. What counts is not the quantity of the exercises performed, but the intensity of the practice. An overdose of yoga philosophy does not increase any effect. It is advisable to read only one or two chapters a day at the most and then practice. By doing so, make time for intensive reflection and contemplation. Like yoga in general, so yoga philosophy feeds on revision. In your physical practice you do not learn a new posture in each lesson, but repeat the same pose over and over and in doing so you gain consciousness and depth. Accordingly, it is better to read one chapter a couple of times and practice, and not work through the chapters superficially one after the other. You might be surprised how in your revision the understanding of the same topic may improve. Thus, the lessons learned from these reflective exercises can be taken into everyday life, and especially when you do not think of them they can suddenly reveal insights and hence unfold their full effective force. The insights of yoga philosophy serve as provisions for everyday life.

Through the practice of yoga philosophy be prepared to take a path that may change you. Yoga philosophy turns into a path once we do not only learn something about yoga, but also about ourselves, about our unconsciousness and our urges, and also about the opportunities to release these in order to get onto a path of more awareness and clarity. Consequently, walking the path of yoga philosophically means to intensify our own way of life, so that we will deepen our awareness about the wonders of life.

I. Historical Backgrounds

1

The Origin of Yoga

What is yoga? Those who have guessed that yoga means a lot more than being able to bend one's body like a pretzel seem to be right, but what does this "more" mean? What is the original meaning of yoga as it was discovered thousands of years ago in ancient India? Interestingly, no one is sure when exactly this discovery took place. In the northwest of the Indian subcontinent in what is nowadays known as Pakistan archeologists dug up city ruins, which probably existed around 3000 BC. In these ruins they found small plaques with images of squatting people, who are reminiscent of yogis sitting on the ground. Yet, being able to remain in a seated posture does not make one a yogi, and looking from an angle of serious research it is not possible to say whether at that time yoga was really known then.

Only later, in the second millennium BC, the oldest Hindu texts originated. These texts speak about "silent ascetics", who had withdrawn from society in order to live a life in complete silence. But can these ascetics, who had withdrawn from the hubbub of everyday life in order to practice silence, really be considered the first yogis?

The real discovery of yoga happened only much later between the 7th and 6th century BC. These first real yogis had little interest in writing down their experiences. However, we are lucky. The priests of that time, the *Brahmans*, recognized the immense value of the discovery of yoga. They integrated the words of the first yogis into their own sacred texts of *Veda* and referred to these earliest texts of yoga with the term *Upanishad*, which means 'secret text'. Many of such secret texts were produced during that time. As the *Upanishads* were not written down, but had to be memorized, they were only delivered orally from teacher to student until they were finally recorded much later in time. Today we have evidence of the origins of yoga in the form of books. Anyone can buy these books so it is no longer necessary, as it used to be, to be a personal student of a *Brahman* or a yoga master in order to learn something about the origins of yoga.

So, what did these first yogis find out when they initially discovered yoga almost 3000 years ago in ancient India? What was written down in the old sacred texts of the *Upanishads*? It is obvious that even in those days it was hard to put yoga experiences into words. However, in order to still be able to explain to their students what they had experienced, these first yogis referred to the concepts of the religion of that time. If we want to understand what yoga means in its original sense, we have to enter the world of the gods of ancient India. We will encounter ancient images that can tell us something important even in today's modern world.

In one of the oldest *Upanishads* three central gods are mentioned: *Indra, Vayu* and *Agni.* These *Vedic* deities had a truly remarkable experience. They met '*brahman*'. The Sanskrit term *brahman* is generally translated to 'the Absolute'. However, the three gods did not recognize *brahman*. The text explains that *brahman* as 'the Absolute' means the foundation of all reality. The universe is based on *brahman.* Not only humans spring from *brahman*, but even the gods themselves are based on *brahman.* Even the most powerful gods live on the power of *brahman*, including *Indra, Vayu* and *Agni.* Initially, these three gods were not aware of *brahman* and thought that they had become gods through their own divine powers. Yet, they noticed that there was something, but they did not recognize it as *brahman* and simply asked themselves: "What marvel is this?"

According to the stories of the *Upanishads* they first sent out *Agni*, the God of Fire, in order to explore this wondrous phenomenon of *brahman.* When *Agni* being aware of his great powers approaches *brahman*, *brahman* turns the tables and asks him: "Who are you?" *Agni* instantly replies that he is the great God of Fire, who could destroy anything that exists in this world. As a test 'the Absolute' then offers *Agni* a straw and asks him to burn it. Strangely, even with the greatest efforts *Agni* did not manage to damage the straw of 'the Absolute' and had to return unsuccessfully to the two other gods.

The second who was sent out was *Vayu*, the God of the Winds. With his great powers he knows how to move anything that exists in air space. 'The Absolute' also offered him a straw, which despite his great powers *Vayu* did not manage to move even a millimeter. He also had to return without success. When in a final trial the king of the gods *Indra* himself tried to explore 'it', 'the Absolute' simply disguised itself to *Indra*. So even with the highest divine force it was not possible to experience the all-establishing reality of 'the Absolute'.

Interestingly, the tale takes the crucial turn exactly at that moment, when all the powers of the gods fail. A completely unknown female character appears, *Uma*, the daughter of *Himalaya*. With her femininity she constitutes a counter pole to the powers of the male gods. *Uma* represents a symbol of surrender, intuition and of 'not doing'. It is this woman who points to the path of letting go and surrender, and who provides the answer to the great gods on their search by explaining: "It is 'the Absolute' on which all your powers are based." Only then does *Indra* first and then the two other gods recognize *brahman*. Now, after they had renounced all of their powers and opened to intuition and surrender, the gods experienced that their lives and powers were not based on their own force, but on the force of *brahman*, 'the Absolute'. They experienced the all-embracing power of 'the Absolute' from which not only humans live, but also the gods themselves.

No exercise is described in any of these oldest texts, neither physical exercises nor breathing exercises nor meditation. No seated yoga postures nor any other yoga postures were known of at that time. Not even the term 'yoga' was known then. In the beginning of yoga there was no practice, but there was an experience. And it was this experience that was sought to be expressed in the philosophy of the *Vedic* religion of that time from which today's Hinduism has developed. It was referred to as the experience of *brahman*, the primal experience from which the entire universe originates without one even being aware of it, and to which man had managed to penetrate for the first time.

Only later the students of these first yogis started to ask for exercises, which could support this primal experience, and so the first yoga exercises were developed.

Although at this time the term 'yoga' was not known, in the images of these oldest texts everything was said that later the various schools of yoga have tried to express in often much more complicated ways. The mighty gods represent all our efforts to lead our lives in our way and to create our lives through doing. For example, if we really put effort into something it is possible to create great wealth and recognition, but even if we were able to arise to gods ourselves in yoga this would not be enough. The first yogis had a truly revolutionary experience. They learnt that there is a reality that even the gods depend on. The path to this experience is expressed in the symbol of *Uma*. *Uma* means letting go. *Uma* means not doing. And this "not doing" is so much more than all the powers and forces in the world of the gods.

The first yogis recognized that man is much more than he can generally perceive. Putting it simply, one could say that the discovery of yoga is the paradoxical experience of 'doing less' and hence 'receiving more'. This 'doing less' is a very peculiar 'doing less'. Yoga encourages a 'doing less' that leads to inner change and to inner detachment, and through this a very special 'receiving more' opens up once man experiences *brahman*, 'the Absolute', in the very depth of his heart in the here and now. If we learn to let go like *Uma* then awareness will break open that in the depth of our hearts we ultimately live out of *brahman*, 'the Absolute'. The origin of yoga points to yoga as a holistic way of life. The origin of yoga points to the discovery of our original and actual divine life.

Exercise

For the following exercise please allow for at least 10 minutes. First, read the entire text and only then start with the exercise of reflection. It is helpful to have a pen and a sheet of paper at hand to be able to jot down the results of each step in keywords.

What is expressed through the male gods, the female Uma and brahman, 'the Absolute', mirrors concrete experiences on the path of yoga. As a first step reflect on moments in your own yoga practice in which you tried to master exercises through 'doing', where you exerted yourself in order to reach your goals and where you had to make an effort to perfect your practice – like the Vedic gods Indra, Vayu and Agni tried to do initially. What are your experiences with this kind of practice?

As a second step look at your practice and identify where you are able to take on Uma's stance and where you can manage to let go.

- *Have you ever managed to surrender to your practice by doing nothing and hence experiencing a force, which carries you without you yourself achieving something?*
- *Can you recall moments in your practice in which you 'do less' in a sense and yet 'receive more'?*

Bring to mind that each yoga practice finds its essence in not you doing the practice, but in the practice carrying you. In the old Upanishads this is expressed in the symbol of Uma.

Perhaps such experiences may give an inkling to what the oldest texts of yoga refer to by the experience of the all-embracing divine power of brahman out of which not only humanity but ultimately the entire reality springs. The origin of yoga points towards experiencing 'the Absolute', which in general we do very seldom. However, from here an inkling of what really matters shines through if we open up to it and surrender.

2

The Three Great Lines of Tradition

In the beginning of the history of yoga was the experience. Students started to gather around the great masters who appeared from the 7th and 6th century BC at the time of the *Upanishads*. The first small yoga circles emerged. Most likely students would ask their masters for ways to find this particular experience. They would ask for exercises that would nurture such experiences. Consequently, meditation was developed as one of the first yoga exercises, partly coupled with preparatory breathing exercises. Yoga also had a strong spiritual focus on the experience of the divine *brahman*. Yoga means a pathway to divine experiences, from where different schools of yoga evolved. These schools understood the yogic path not as a religious one, but rather as a philosophical one. For these more philosophically oriented schools meditation also evolved to be the central practice. However, here the practice was directed towards the experience of the 'highest Self'. This 'Self' – an experience of the innermost center of man – is described with the Sanskrit term *atman*. Yoga was seen as a path towards awareness for the deepest essence of man. From these schools a second line of tradition emerged: the classical-philosophical yoga. Hence, for a long time it was possible to distinguish between two basic forms of yoga, one with a strong religious focus and the other with a more philosophical focus. In both forms of yoga meditation played a crucial part, on the one hand coupled with rituals of surrender and religious-meditative chanting, and on the other hand with philosophical reflection.

Only later in time, perhaps from the 10th or 11th century AD, a third line of tradition emerged, when it was discovered that it is particularly helpful to integrate the body into the practice. This was the great hour of *hatha yoga*, the yoga that integrates physical exercises into the practice.

If today's yoga presents itself in a variety of ways of practice, directions, names and personalities and can look back on a nearly 3000 year old history, all of these yogic pathways are ultimately based on the three great lines of tradition: first the religious yoga, second the philosophical yoga and third *hatha yoga*, which integrates physical exercise. These three lines of tradition each have their own basic texts, theories and even their own terminology. When today's schools of yoga refer to these three lines of tradition, they do so with very differing focuses. Some schools have their central focus on the pathway of religious yoga, others focus on classical-philosophical yoga and others on *hatha yoga*.

In this chapter, these three lines of tradition will be introduced briefly. First, the 'religious yoga': The primal experience of yoga was the experience of *brahman*, 'the Absolute'. The first yoga exercise of meditation was understood to be a pathway for divine experience, and the *Upanishads*, the oldest texts, which describe all this, are still honored as sacred texts by Hindus today. Thus, religious yoga refers to religion, but must not be confused as religion itself. The religious language, religious beliefs or religious rituals only constitute to the beginning or an outer sheath of this yoga. By entering the path of yoga the concept of religion begins to transform. Within religious yoga the belief of an external god outside humans continually evolves to the experience of the Divine residing deeply inside humans. An externally directed focus on the words of a priest or the commandments and teachings of the sacred texts transforms into the believer's surrender to the depth of his very own existence. Meditation, sacrifice and religious chanting especially turn into a practice of inner transformation, to a point where all 'I-ness' is dissolved and where the yogi lives alone out of a divine experience from the very depths of his innermost center. Various religious texts on yoga emerged, of which the *Bhagavadgita* stands out especially. The *Bhagavadgita* is worshiped as the most important sacred text by many Hindus, and at the same time is considered the most significant text of religious yoga. Today nearly all yoga centers in India include the practice of meditative chanting and recitation of religious yoga.

The idea that the path of yoga can have religion at its source, but does not need to, can be seen in the second great line of tradition, the 'classical-philosophical yoga'. This yoga is based on the *Yoga Sutras* of *Patañjali*, which are believed to date back to between the 2nd century BC and the 2nd century AD. In a sort of compendium *Patañjali* analyzes what happens inside the human when he practices yoga. He explains the state of consciousness that the practitioner starts, the kinds of transformations and changes that take place during the practice, and what the perspective of the yogic experience is. *Patañjali* also develops the famous Eightfold Path of Yoga in which the principles of nonreligious yoga meditation are introduced. In the times thereafter his *Yoga Sutras* became *the* fundamental texts on yoga per se. Numerous commentaries appeared, which modified the classical-philosophical yoga. Consequently, anyone who has looked into yoga within the past 2000 years in some way or another draws on the *Yoga Sutras* as a source.

Hatha yoga, the youngest line of tradition, which emerged at the start of the 2nd millennium AD, also draws on *Patañjali*. To be precise *hatha yoga* is actually not a separate line of tradition, but rather a big integration movement of yoga. *Hatha yoga* is based on religious yoga as well as on classical-philosophical yoga, and integrates physical exercises into these more mind-related practices. Hence, the body is discovered as a gate for enlightenment, and only much later was the physical practice of *hatha yoga*, that is so popular today, developed and practiced alongside numerous breathing exercises.

For several centuries *hatha yoga* experienced its heydays until together with all other forms of yoga it was buried in oblivion.

The degradation of India to a British colony in the modern era added to the downfall of yoga. Only in the 20th century a recollection of its own cultural heritage started to evolve and with this a new look on yoga emerged. Great yogis like *Vivekananda, Aurobindo, Yogananda* or *Ramana Maharshi* rediscovered the old treasures of yoga and began to make yoga available for the modern Indian, but also for the interested Westerner. However, these yogis exclusively referred to the traditions of religious and classical-philosophical yoga. Then, the yogic masters, who in addition began to teach *hatha yoga*, became the most successful as the physical exercises were adapted enthusiastically by Western students. This has led to the yoga boom that we experience today in the West.

This glance at the great history of yoga shows that yoga is much more than just physical exercise. Yoga is diverse and manifold, and thus offers a chance to find your own yogic path that suits your personality. Moreover, various types of exercises can be combined in order to support one's own way of life. However, the following analogy reminds us to be cautious: If we look for water here one day and there another, we may not be able to dig very deep. It is better to find the right spot and dig deeply with passion and persistence. Consequently, it is important to go deep, but to do so at the right spot. Then we will not only find water, but we will have the chance to discover the true treasures of yoga.

Exercise

Take a few minutes and contemplate where within the broad spectrum of the three lines of tradition you have already 'dug for water'?

- *Have you already been in touch with religious yoga? Do you know the practice of religious meditation or have you come across meditative chanting and recitation?*
- *Have you already been in touch with the classical-philosophical yoga, the nonreligious yoga meditation or with the famous Eightfold Path of Yoga by Patañjali?*
- *Or is your focus on hatha yoga, which integrates the body into the practice?*

Numerous exercises have been developed in the nearly three thousand year old history of yoga, all of which serve as aids to dig deeply in order to find the hidden treasure of our true Self. It is important, however, to dig at the right spot.

Finally ask yourself:

- *Have you found the right form of practice for yourself yet?*
- *Or do you find it necessary to keep on searching and try other forms of practice from the broad field of the yoga traditions?*

If you are getting the notion that your form of practice is the right one for you, then it is worthwhile to put energy and persistence into it in order to truly go deeply, in order to 'find water' and to discover the abundance of yoga as a source. Only through 'digging deeply', that is an intensive practice, will it be possible to grow in yoga in order to find the virtually undreamed of treasures of yoga.

II. The Yogic Pathway

3

The Way Inside

Since ancient times the practice of Hinduism has been characterized by sacrificial cult, worship and prayer, through which the believers thanked a god or deities, or they may have asked for help and protection. When 'the Divine' was discovered *inside* humans, the practice took a crucial turn, at least for those who made this discovery. The primordial experience of yoga as the experience of *brahman*, 'the Absolute', *in* humans constituted a revolution. The question of god now appeared to be closely related to the question of humanity. The gaze to the gods no longer turned upwards, towards the heavens, but changed to a path inside. Likewise, the concept of the nature of human beings changed essentially. It was discovered that human beings are much more than just beings of body and mind.

In an old image from the *Upanishads* man is described as "the City of God", in which there is a small house like that of a lotus flower. What is to be found in this deepest 'inside' is to be explored. Since ancient times the lotus has been a symbol of the inner liberation of man, of a divine freedom, which cannot be lived in the consciousness of everyday life. Normally, man lives outside of 'his city', outside of himself. Consciousness faces towards the outside. In the language of yoga the senses are linked to the sense objects. Man only recognizes the surface of his opportunities and is constrained by outer circumstances and by encountered implicitness. He is driven by his aspirations for wealth, recognition and the satisfaction of his desires. Yet, deep inside man there lies an undiscovered treasure. So how is it possible to free oneself from all the daily constraints in order to enter 'the City of God' and thereby one's true Self? Yoga provides the answer as a way inside.

The first step on this path is to reverse the course of the outwardly consciousness. The first step means a withdrawal from everyday life. Like a tortoise retracts its limbs, so a yogi withdraws the senses from the sense objects when he starts his practice, making it important to find a quiet space for the practice away from everyday turmoil and the various distractions. In such a place of tranquility it will be easier to find stillness and to not be distracted by visual or auditory stimuli of the environment. This first step of sense withdrawal forms a foundation for each following step.

Likewise, one has to penetrate one sheath after another on the way inside and on the search for the inner center of the true, divine Self. Thus, it needs to be recognized that the material body breathes, is alive and is carried by life force. Going further inside, the yogi experiences that he is not only matter and life force, but also has a psyche to think and feel with. From here it becomes feasible to become aware of the outer coarser sheaths of body and mind.

Yet, the path of yoga goes even deeper inside. The sheath of the psyche also needs to be penetrated and be opened up for the experience of inner, intuitive knowledge. Intuitive knowledge emerges once one manages to open up for an inner awareness beyond thought. This also means that opening for this inner dimension cannot be done or created. From here on the practice of 'doing less' becomes effective, so that the sheath of intuitive knowing can be experienced. Yet, it is only a sheath for an even deeper dimension to come.

The one who has managed to go beyond unconsciousness and darkness, and in this way has managed to penetrate through thought and intuitive knowledge, then may be able to experience a form of joy, that is not created from outside. In order to differentiate this inner, immediate joy from outer experiences of happiness, it is mostly referred to as 'bliss', the 'sheath of bliss'.

Yet again, it is only a sheath. This 'bliss sheath' needs to be penetrated further, in order to reach the innermost essence of human existence, which is traditionally referred to as *brahman*, 'the Absolute', the divine nature of man. The one who has managed to penetrate this deeply into the innermost center is able to experience a force that really carries in this world. He has managed to awaken to his inner essence and to his original state of being human, which is so much more than one would have ever thought. In this innermost center one experiences his original union with *brahman*, 'the Absolute'. Only now may it become conceivable what the early yogis meant, when they referred to man as 'a City of God', in which there is a small house like that of a lotus flower.

Exercise

The sheath model offers wonderful opportunities to comprehend the yogic way inside step by step. For the following exercise first find a place of quietude and then start to withdraw your senses from the outside to the inside like a tortoise withdraws its limbs. That is do not look around or listen to what is happening in the room next door, but focus your inner gaze on yourself and go inside.

- *First, feel your body starting with the feet, knees, thighs, your buttocks, your tummy, back, neck, shoulders, your arms until you have reached your fingers and finally your head and crown.*
- *Second, go a step further inside. Experience that your body is breathing. Experience how you inhale and exhale. Become aware of how your body feeds from your inner life force and that you are alive.*
- *The next step will take you further inside. Feel your psyche, your thoughts and how they are connected to your feelings, needs and desires. Feel this third sheath and how you can perceive the other sheaths, your life and your body from here. These initial stages on your journey inside should be quite feasible.*

From here on the crucial opening for the primal inner experience, that which makes yoga yoga, can happen. To go even deeper inside from here means to 'do less' and to finally 'not do' anymore. This is the deeper purpose of the physical exercises, the breathing exercises and also of yoga meditation. Stay in this open awareness of the inside, where you are focused, yet relaxed, and hence can open up to your innermost centeredness.

In the following reflection look back on the various stages of your way inside.

- *Become aware that by doing less, deeper and deeper sheaths of your existence can open up, until finally the undiscovered treasure of your inner essence may begin to unfold.*

Only now may it become conceivable what the early yogis of the Upanishads meant, when they called man 'a City of God', in which there is a small house like that of a lotus flower.

4

The Beginning – The Ties of Everyday Consciousness

Now, what does the path that the great masters of yoga have discovered look like? Yoga encourages a change in awareness. What is this change like? Where does it begin? What is the process? Where does it lead to? In order to understand what yoga does with us, it is important to go back a long way in the process of the beginning of our consciousness. All humans develop a consciousness within the first years of their lives. Through our consciousness we become aware that there is a world and in this world there is us. However, with this great accomplishment of humanity there comes a fundamental problem. The world and all life in it are constrained by time. Everything passes. Sensual pleasures, gathered wealth, recognition by the ones around us, our friends and lastly we ourselves pass.

The problem herein does not lie in the awareness of the impermanence of the world. The problem is that in our everyday consciousness, which has created over time, we do identify with this transitory world. We have distanced ourselves from our true Self, and identify with all those fading objects of this world. We are attached to them, but ultimately this attachment is futile. All our sensual pleasures, our wealth and our recognition will fade. And each time we experience loss, there will be suffering.

Yet, we do not experience suffering only. We have developed mechanisms in our everyday consciousness that compensate for the suffering of impermanence through the creation of an outer stability. The Indian tradition names three of these stabilizing factors concerning everyday consciousness. The first one is 'repression' of all suffering. If man does not recognize that all his wealth and all his pleasures will pass and if he does not recognize the impermanence in this world, then he also denies the suffering in all passing. This repression works as long as man believes that 'one' dies and as long as this 'one' refers to the others, but not to himself.

Secondly, the ordinary 'I' is not only stabilized through unconsciousness, but also through a constant search for outer states of happiness. We seek happiness through a constant satisfaction of our desires, for example through gathering even greater wealth, through a need of recognition and rewards from successful actions. All these factors only create an outer and impermanent happiness. Yet, this kind of happiness continuously manages to compensate for the sufferings in the world and stabilizes the ego of our everyday consciousness.

A third factor in this context is the belief that this ever changing, impermanent world is yet held together through an eternal 'order'. This is expressed in the belief in laws, according to which everything works, or divine commandments that say what is good and right. Religious doctrines as well as today's belief in the omnipotence of modern science enable us to identify directions and a goal in the impermanence of this world.

Whether man chooses repression, a life that aims to satisfy sensual pleasures or prefers to find stability in a belief system with eternal laws within a fixed world order, these three enable us to gain balance and find stability in a fundamentally impermanent world. However, this everyday consciousness eventually becomes unstable. Crises will appear when steadiness breaks away, but such crises can be overcome. Some repetitively go for repression, some for more sex, wealth or professional success, and others reinforce their belief that there is the one truth. Again and again, one may be able to succeed in carrying on in the old ways and not having to change. We can indeed remain in this state of everyday consciousness up to our last days, and most people do so.

Nevertheless, what started with the discovery of yoga constitutes a revolution. Most people when making their way onto their yoga mat are not quite aware of the revolutionary path they have just entered. Yoga is about untying the bondages that our ego of everyday consciousness appreciates so much. Because of these ties man has forgotten to be aware of his true Self. In his constant search for renewed happiness through recognition, sexual satisfaction or praise from others man runs past himself. The belief in a set of doctrines, which state what is right or wrong, has been unmasked as heteronomy. As such everyday consciousness is compared to a boat that is swept away by the wind:

When the mind follows the roaming senses, these carry away man's consciousness, just as a wind sweeps away a boat on the water.
(Bhagavadgita 2.67)

We are all like a sailing boat in open waters. At times there is a slack. Then we drift unconsciously on the waters of our lives. At other times the wind of outer happiness blows. These are the 'roaming senses' that sweep away our boat on the waters. In everyday consciousness man thinks that he is in control of his own life. Yet, he is not able to see how he is drifting here and there on the open waters of life, depending on the direction from which the winds of our addictions to outer happiness blow. As long as we believe ourselves to be in control, there is no need to change. As long as we believe that the tensions in our body are a foothold, we will nourish and cherish them. Likewise as long as an externally encountered doctrine provides a foothold we will cling to its truth.

For most people there is hardly a need to enter the path of yoga, because in everyday consciousness there are manifold ways to counterbalance the sufferings of the world. Why then should we start yoga? Yoga becomes interesting once our everyday footholds begin to crumble. This could start with never-ending insomnia or with back pains that continuously become worse. Finally, one may even develop the desire to radically change something in one's life. Only when our experiences of outer happiness cannot counterbalance the basic sufferings of impermanence any longer, the search for experiences of inner happiness will get under way. Only when the binding footholds of sacred teachings turn into constricting cuffs, a desire for freedom and liberation from these cuffs of hardened teachings may appear; and only once we realize that we are not the master on board our own boat, but that we are swept away by outer winds, like a boat without a master on open waters, only then does the deeper meaning of yoga become truly relevant for us.

What happens next is expressed in the popular image of the snake and the rope:

A rope appears as a snake as long as our illusion lasts. Once the illusion ends, the existence of the snake ends.
(Shankara: The Crest Jewel of Discrimination)

In the darkness a rope can easily be mistaken as a snake. In the darkness of our everyday consciousness we are unaware of how tied down and trapped we are. We assume that we actually are the way we have become. But therein lies a fundamental illusion. The rope is a rope and not a snake. What is meant is that we have distanced ourselves from our true Self. We are tied down, driven and trapped, and finally we are no longer ourselves. If there was light, we could see that the snake was not a snake, but a rope. If we were to awaken to our primal consciousness we could recognize who we truly are. Once on the yogic path we no longer need to wait for outside help, for someone who turns on the light of our consciousness. With the practices of yoga we have oppor-tunities at hand to work on our own transformation. All yogic exercises support the process of our awakening, the growing awareness for our inner center. Yoga supports illumination. It unties the bondages of body and mind, so that we can return to our Self and awaken to who we truly are.

Exercise

In the following exercise take a look at yourself. In your life what is it that provides for stability, a foothold and direction? According to the three factors mentioned in the Indian tradition, which of these can you identify with?

- *Do unconsciousness, denial and repression determine your life?*
- *Or does a search for outer happiness, the satisfaction of sensual pleasures, gathering wealth, a focus on successful action provide meaning and stability for you?*
- *Or have you found a foothold in a belief system that is true for you?*

Secondly, reflect on experiences where this stability has started to crumble.

- *Do you know the experience of being swept away like a boat on open waters? Bring to mind situations where you were driven in such manner.*
- *Are you familiar with experiences of being tied down or driven, when you are not yourself any longer? How do you experience yourself in such moments?*
- *Have you ever had an experience where the stability of your everyday consciousness has started to crumble? What are such situations?*
- *Have you experienced yet that such stability can be an illusion, like the alleged snake in the darkness that is actually a rope?*

Now, think of these experiences as by no means bad ones concerning the yogic path, but consider that they can be the crucial reason to embark on a journey in order to change something.

- *What have you done so far in order to undo the obscuring ties and urges of your everyday consciousness?*

5

The Pathway – Transformation of Body and Mind

Yoga means change, transformation of body and mind. How does this transformation happen? How does yoga change the practitioner? One of the most important definitions of the yogic transformational process can be found in *Patañjali's Yoga Sutras*, the most significant text of classical-philosophical yoga. If we ask ourselves, what is going to happen when we make our way onto the mat in order to practice yoga, *Patañjali's* answer is: '*nirodha*'. *Nirodha* means 'calming down the active mind', but in yoga what are the benefits of calming down? It is our active mind, or to be more precise the attachments of our active mind, which represent our urging thoughts, feelings, needs or desires, all the inner activities, which we perceive when we close our eyes and start to observe ourselves. What is peculiar about this mind is that we are not in charge of its activities. Thoughts come and go without us being able to influence their coming and going. Situations or people wind us up, thoughts and feelings appear inside of us, whether we like them or not. Needs and desires emerge and begin to drive and determine us. However, ultimately these attachments are not only limited to mind and soul. Also, tensions or cramping pains in our body come and go and we may not be in control of them.

Consequently, yoga means a process of transforming body and mind through dissolving ties and bondages. Tensions in body and mind begin to disappear. Less often are we driven by our active mind of needs and desires, hence it will loosen its binding power.

What *Patañjali* expressed rather abstractly in one single term *nirodha*, calming down the mind, can be found in one of the old

Upanishads in a wonderful image. In it the process of yogic transformation is described as "undoing all ties that are knitted around the human heart." In the Indian tradition the heart is not only the home of our emotions, but also of the mind. In everyday consciousness our heart has many ties knotted around it. Feelings and thoughts are bound, have hardened, perhaps they are even tense and thus obscure our innermost center. The pathway of yoga means to undo these knots around the heart and to dissolve our inner tightness. When we loosen the knots around our heart, we are freeing our inner center. The clarity of our awareness coming from the heart increases.

Another common comparison of this yogic process of transformation is the image of cleansing muddy waters. Body and mind are compared to waters which are polluted by the muds of tensions, addictions or emotional ties. Driven by thoughts and emotions we are not ourselves. Hence, it is impossible to see the bottom of our innermost center nor to live from there.

But how can we clean these muddy waters so that we can see the bottom? What can we do to calm down our active mind, so that the knots around our hearts begin to loosen? Any attempt to remove the mud by hand or by using a tool bears the risk to move the water and stir up more mud. Any attempt to remove tensions by putting effort into them will only suppress and harden them. Consequently, we have to wait for the mud to settle. Eventually, the water does the cleaning itself, and likewise all yoga exercises aim to practice 'doing nothing' or at least they practice 'letting go' and 'doing less'.

Of course, practice means activity. However, the individual activity is only the beginning. As long as the practice is an effort we are still beginners. The further we progress in our practice, the less we will be 'doing'. As such the motto is 'doing less and receiving more in return'. Hence, somehow the path of yoga seems completely illogical and contradicts our everyday consciousness, which commonly says 'do more and consequently receive more'. From early childhood on we are taught: "Do your homework and you will receive good marks in school." Calming our active mind, however, works quite differently and is comparable to the image of clearing muddy waters. Yoga begins to work when we learn to do less, but yoga refers to a very specific 'doing less'. Here, doing less does not mean to lean back and drift. Rather, it is about a concentrated letting go. Growing in practice means to do less and less, and to be increasingly carried by a force from the inner center, and this force cannot be 'made'. Our busy mind begins to calm down, and the ties and knots around the heart begin to loosen. The impurities of the tensions of our body and mind slowly dissolve. Inner clarity and strength will grow and we begin to experience being carried by a life from our inner center. When practicing yoga, what we call the yogic transformational process becomes evidently experiential, and that is the calming of the busy mind or this very particular 'doing less'. However, in order to experience this, generally a long and consistent yoga practice is required.

Exercise

In the following exercise bring to mind to what extent your yoga practice is still a 'doing'.

- *To what extent is your practice difficult or tedious and requires an effort?*
- *In your yoga class do you often compare yourself to your neighbors or check if they do everything right?*
- *Or do you rather align yourself according to the perfect poses as they are shown in yoga books?*
- *Hence, to what extent can your practice be described as 'doing'?*

Each yoga practice begins with effort and 'doing' and with the alignment towards an external ideal. Over time, however, and all by itself the practice will begin to open for the particular yogic way of 'not doing'.

- *Go on a search and reflect whether your practice has changed over time. Have you experienced the yogic transformational process yourself yet?*
- *Have you experienced 'doing less and getting more in return' yet when your practice is flowing and when a great force of lightness is emerging?*
- *Have you ever experienced that clarity of body and mind can come to the surface when the muds of our tensions and urges begin to settle?*
- *Have you ever had the feeling of inner liberation?*
- *Have you ever had the experience of being carried by a higher force that you did not 'make' or 'produce'?*

Take time to bring these experiences to mind and explore them. These are experiences of calming down the busy mind, which can be expressed in the term nirodha. This calming down of all addictions and urges enables us to grow in our yoga practice and to awaken us to our true Self.

6

The Destination – Awakening to Our True Self

Yoga is looking for a treasure and we ourselves are this treasure. We are detached from our true Selves and yoga can bring us back. Yet, we are a lot more than we generally assume and much more than we could make or produce. Hence, the path to our true Selves does not involve a 'doing', but it is a practice, in which we learn in a very specific way to do less and less in order to receive more, and in order to discover who we truly are. Finally, the perspective is a 'not doing' all together in order to experience everything, that is our Self, our true Self.

However, usually treasures are buried or at least they lie hidden somewhere, and so the treasure of yoga is buried. The treasure of our true Self is hidden deeply inside of us and is waiting to be discovered. This concealment of the true Self is expressed vividly in the following quote from one of the *Upanishads*:

As there is oil in sesame, butter in milk, water in underground springs and fire in firewood, so the one who searches in truthfulness and practice will realize the true Self inside himself.
(Shvetashvatara Upanishad 1.16)

What is man? When is man himself? Everyday consciousness only touches the surface. Man's existence, however, reaches much deeper. The superficial existence of the everyday consciousness is compared to a sesame seed, in which the oil is hidden invisibly inside and yet it is there. Like the oil in the sesame seed, the true Self of man is invisible from unconscious viewing. Another comparison describes our superficiality as milk. The butter is invisibly hidden inside the milk like the actual

Self in us. The same applies to water hidden in underground springs or fire, which cannot be seen in firewood.

Being on the path of yoga means to go on a search for the hidden true Self inside of us. Practicing yoga enables a breakthrough to our Selves, but only if practiced genuinely. It is like making fire from firewood, when after drilling for a long time, it appears as if we are not doing anything and the drilling just happens by itself. Then, all of a sudden there is a spark of fire, and all by itself the veil of everyday consciousness begins to lift.

The destination of yoga lies in this breakthrough, which can be called 'enlightenment' or 'awakening', an awakening from the sleep of our unconsciousness. Looking back from here the axiomatic ties of our everyday consciousness appear like a dream, a dream in which we were incapable to actually lead our lives. As long as we are dreaming, we believe our dreams to be the reality. As long as we live in everyday consciousness we assume our unconsciousness to be completely normal. We don't know anything else than being driven by our thoughts and emotions or being addicted to our desires or to the acknowledgements from our fellow men. We believe these to be our reality. The everyday consciousness seems immutable. Only through an awakening it becomes feasible to realize that all our previous thoughts and emotions have only formed the surface of our existence. We awaken and we begin to realize what really counts and who we truly are. We recognize our true Self as the deeply hidden treasure in order to be able to live from the depths of our very own existence.

Only the one who has experienced the Self can comprehend what treasure is to be discovered in yoga. For this reason, it is repeatedly stressed that the highest yogic experience cannot be put into words. Yet, there have been continuous attempts to verbalize these experiences. In the *Upanishads* the experience of 'the Absolute', *brahman*, is emphasized; or similarly the experience of the true Self, *atman*. At the times of the classical-philosophical yoga of the *Yoga Sutras* by *Patañjali* the Sanskrit term *samadhi* emerged as the central term for the transcendental experiences of yoga. *Samadhi* can be translated literally to 'oneness'. Some ascetics, however, who considered yoga to be a path of worldly rejection, mistook *samadhi* as a state of immersion, in which the human mind was believed to have to escape into certain ulterior realms. Some yogis even let themselves be buried for days in holes in the ground in deeply immersed states of consciousness and thought themselves to be in *samadhi*. The perspective of yoga is not quite as spectacular as this, but it incorporates a lot more than anything that could impress some simple minds in a sensational show like this.

A famous image from the *Hatha Yoga Pradipika*, the most important text of *hatha yoga*, portrays who or what man becomes 'one' with when he awakens to the state of *samadhi*.

Like a grain of salt dissolves in water, so the mind becomes one with the highest Self. This is samadhi, the highest union of all.
(*Hatha Yoga Pradipika*, 4.5)

Like a grain of salt dissolves in water, we dissolve in our highest Self. What does this mean when we dissolve? And who dissolves? What is this grain of salt? The grain of salt is our everyday consciousness. Our tensions and tightness in body and mind begin to vanish, and so do our fixed thought patterns and our emotional blindness. Just like a grain of salt dissolves in water, our dependences on people, who wind us up or make us jealous, dissolve. Also, the attachments to external happiness, such as good food, sex or recognition from others begin to loosen. Our mock appearance of our everyday consciousness begins to dissipate, so that we can awaken to an inner union with our true Self. The unconsciousness of everyday life does not enable us to live from this place, yet we can return to be one with the Self, as was the case originally.

Exercise

Of course many, especially those at the beginning of the yogic path, will ask themselves what to do with this perspective of yoga as enlightenment and awakening. Most of us can only experience sparks of enlightenment, the very first effects of yoga. Yet, for more than 3000 years all texts on yoga have referred to this all-encompassing experience of awakening. The great Indian masters of yoga also point towards enlightenment in the sense of awakening to our true Self as the perspective of yoga, but how can we deal with this vast perspective in today's life?

Please ask yourself the following three questions:

- *What thoughts cross your mind when you read of divine experiences, 'oneness' in samadhi or awakening to the true Self?*
- *Considering this perspective of yoga, which looks at such an enormous treasure, are you rather indifferent about it, do you find it deterring or are you embracing it?*
- *How can dealing with such a wide perspective be beneficial for your current yoga practice?*
- *Find at least one thought or impulse that can be helpful and serve as provision on your future practical yoga journey.*

Before you continue to read, give yourself sufficient time to ponder on these central questions of yoga philosophy in order to get clear answers for yourself.

7

Living in Freedom in the World

All yoga exercises point towards a path inside. The practitioners begin to withdraw from the turmoil of everyday life. They stop engaging once here and once there, but begin to redirect their attention inwards towards the body and the breath, and to any processes that are connected to this withdrawal. Yoga meditation puts an even stronger emphasis on this inward turn. Hence, some have concluded that yoga is a withdrawal from the world. Even the *Bhagavadgita*, which was written some 2000 years ago, describes this common misunderstanding of yoga as worldly withdrawal. One can read about a yogic ascetic who withdrew into meditation and had left everything behind, even his beloved wife, children, wealth and social recognition. While sitting in pride because he believed himself to be on the yogic path due to his withdrawal, all he could do was to constantly dwell on what he had left behind: his wife, children, wealth and social status. This yogi did not understand what was meant by yoga. He withdrew from outer worldly activities into solitude, and yet internally he was still emotionally and mentally attached to all the things he loved.

This alleged yogi thought that yoga means to detach from all activity and withdraw from the world. However, the *Bhagavadgita* strongly emphasizes that everyone, and consequently every human being practicing yoga, can never stop engaging in this world as long as he is still in his physical body. Wherever man goes he takes himself and the world with him. The yogi, who withdraws into a cave in the *Himalayas* or into a room in a yoga center, simply swaps one place in the world for another. But what is significant here is that he has always stayed the same. Yoga does not mean to change the place but to change the person, not through external modifications but through an inner transformation.

Certainly, it can be very useful to withdraw from everyday turmoil into silent solitude to enable this internal transformation, but this external withdrawal is always only preparation, never the final destination. A withdrawal into silence is a preparation for inner stillness, which later on can be lived in the turmoil of everyday life. In yogic serenity, dependences on external influences and manipulations disintegrate. One becomes free of the attachments to a constant search for recognition, to the urges from desires and to simply drifting along unconsciously.

In order to fully understand the meaning of detachment in everyday life, the *Bhagavadgita* refers to the popular image of the lotus flower. Man behaves like a lotus flower in water. The lotus has its roots in the muddy grounds of a pond, but the flower sits on the surface of the water without being wet by it. Like the lotus is rooted in the mud and its petals stay completely pristine, so a real yogi is able to live in the mundane world and yet is not attached to worldly matters any longer. He is able to engage in the unrest of everyday life and yet is not moved by it.

The path towards a detachment of 'ties' and 'bondages' is also portrayed in another image of the *Bhagavadgita* as the image of a candle in the wind. In the beginning mind and psyche behave like an open flame flickering in the wind. The mind is fickle like a flame in the wind when searching for recognition, more wealth or renewed happiness through the satisfaction of desires. One is attached, and hence tied down and dependent.

Yoga, however, is a life in freedom in the midst of the world, and this freedom can only be experienced through inner stability, which enables a detachment from worldly matters. So, the advanced mind behaves like a sheltered flame inside a lamp. This flame does not flicker any longer, but is calm and steady; and likewise, despite a turbulent world the yogi is able to stay steady within. The path of yogic practice begins with turning inside and thus enables us to become aware of the inner center. This experience of inner centeredness must be lived in a life from the force of the true Self, from the force of 'the Divine' in freedom in the world.

Exercise

Bring to mind the two images of the lotus flower in a pond and the flame inside a lamp. Now do not look at these images as some fascinating allegories of a yogi's life, but instead as the images of your own life. Imagine you are a lotus flower sitting in the middle of a big pond, your life. Your roots reach to the bottom of the pond. These roots anchor you in the midst of a turbulent world. Perhaps your life involves a partner, children, a job, wealth or other things that are dear to you. Your flower sits on the surface of the water, but your petals are not wet by the waters of everyday life. Perhaps you can identify with this image only partly or not at all. However, this image is only a yogic ideal and under no circumstances the reality of our lives yet.

The path towards this ideal is also portrayed in captivating clarity in the image of the open flame of a candle. Bring to mind any situations where your life is flickering like a candle in the wind. Become aware of situations in which you are attached to worldly matters, when you are torn by external forces or when you let yourself be torn. What are the things that tie you down?

- *Perhaps it is the need for recognition through others, success in your job or family life?*
- *Or is it the joy of your belongings and pride that you have managed to create or achieve something?*
- *Or are you bound to sex, good food or the satisfaction of your desires?*

Inside a lampshade the candle's flame stops flickering. It stays calm in any kind of weather. In your life have you had experiences of such inner stillness? Bring to mind situations in which you have experienced inner stability, when you are calm and centered, and when you can live from the stability of this true Self in the midst of any worldly turmoil.

- *For example, have you ever experienced that you were offended or insulted and you did not automatically turn to the ties of aggression and anger, but managed to stay calmly centered in your Self like a steady flame inside a lamp?*
- *Have you ever experienced yourself in hectic situations of everyday life, where everyone else was driven by attachments or outer forces, but you could find yourself unmoved, because you were able to find stillness through an inner force?*

Any experience of agitation shows us the importance of a continuous practice. Any experience of inner stability shows us the effects of our consistent practice. On the mat we are practicing to support experiences of inner stability, and when we leave the mat this practice does not cease. Then, the perspective of yoga to live freely in the midst of any upheaval in everyday life begins to open up.

III. The Philosophy of Practice

8

The Nature of Yoga Practice

In the nearly 3000 year old tradition of yoga a virtually immeasurable variety of practices has evolved. The physical exercises of the *asanas* are widely known today. Some of the oldest practices are the breathing exercises of *pranayama* as well as meditation. *Karma yoga*, the yoga of action, *bhakti yoga*, the yoga of religious devotion and *jnana yoga*, the yoga of philosophy are also part of the great classical lines of yoga practice. But within such a great variety of yogic pathways, what is the all-encompassing connecting principle? What criteria are relevant to turn a practice into a yogic practice?

What all practices have in common is the task of cleansing body and mind. In an old image all tensions, the unconsciousness and our addictions are compared to the dust sitting on a mirror. Other images use clouds, smoke or fog, which hinder the sun of our true Self to shine through. The yoga practice then works like a piece of cloth or like brushes that clean the mirror. Yoga enables a dispersion of the inner clouds, so that awareness for the depths of our true Self can emerge.

How does a yoga practice manage to achieve such effects? How does yoga work? Yoga has frequently been misunderstood in parts or even completely. In ancient India there was a jeopardizing tendency to achieve an inner cleansing of the unconsciousness and addictions through external austerity. From the outside it appeared that the ascetic had given up everything, but on the inside the mirror of his mind remained polluted and obscured through his dependences on things.

In today's Western cultures a very differing misunderstanding can be noticed, when a yoga practice is reduced to physical practice only in order to increase levels of achievements

55

and fitness. A yoga practice helps to train certain abilities such as being able to hold extreme postures or the breath for a long time, and these exercises can yield impressive effects. Yet, this is not necessarily yoga in the sense of an inner cleansing. Neither through traditional ascetic mortification nor through a modern body cult will it become possible to disperse the clouds of our unconsciousness in order to let the sun of the true Self shine through.

In order to understand what turns our practice into a *yoga* practice, it is useful to look at the great classical scriptures of yoga, the *Yoga Sutras* by *Patañjali*. The *Yoga Sutras* list two main principles. These two principles are called *abhyasa* and *vairagya* in Sanskrit and can be translated to 'practice' and 'non-attachment'. *Abhyasa* and *vairagya* are two principles that belong together like the two sides of a medal. Only if it becomes feasible to realize both of them, yoga becomes yoga. Practice and non-attachment are the two criteria that tell us whether our practice is truly yoga, whether there is only gymnastics and body building on the one hand, only relaxation and wellness on the other.

The first principle *abhyasa* means 'practice' and refers to active doing and the specific efforts of the practitioner. Especially in the beginning *abhyasa* is very important. It is about actively getting ready for the path and to develop a practice, to focus on body and breath, but also on the sound of a *mantra* in meditation for example. That is practice. However, if the focus in yoga is only on *abhyasa* and hence on effort and concentration, there may be the risk that tensions of our everyday consciousness will increase. They will not dissolve, but on the contrary intensify. In an extreme case such a practice will become a forced practice.

Thus, in genuine yoga *abhyasa* is always linked to the practice of *vairagya*, the non-attachment to any efforts and endeavors. In *vairagya* the practitioner is passive. In *vairagya* the practitioner lets go of all doing and of all efforts, and here one experiences relaxation, a flow or surrender. This does not mean that yoga is only letting go and relaxation. To overemphasize detachment will lead to aimless drifting and fruitless idleness. The everyday consciousness will remain in its accustomed structures without any change.

If yoga was only *abhyasa*, that is practice, endurance and effort, one could only achieve what is doable. If on the other hand one only practices *vairagya*, that is non-attachment, body and mind would drift without awareness.

What is special in practicing yoga is the connection of *abhyasa* and *vairagya*, of active effort and concentration and passive letting go and relaxation. From the perspective of everyday consciousness this may sound controversial. How can one be active and passive at the same time? If it was so easy, one did not need to practice yoga persistently and over a long period of time. It is normal to continuously veer off to one side or the other when practicing, but once practice and non-attachment are combined a very particular form of activeness and passiveness will emerge. The practice becomes focused and yet serene and relaxed. The kind of 'doing less' emerges, in which one can 'receive more'. Practice and non-attachment can merge once the practitioner begins to do less and lets himself be carried increasingly. In merging *abhyasa* and *vairagya* the experience of a force of lightness awakens. This force of lightness can be experienced in body, in mind, in breath, in everyday living and also in religious rituals. I begin to do less and receive more and more. And finally I do nothing but receive everything.

This points towards the idea that practicing yoga is not an end in itself. The practice works towards exercising less and less to finally even leaving the practice itself behind. An allegory from the *Upanishads* states:

A cart is only of service as long as there is a road. The one who reaches the end of the road then dismounts and walks.
(Amritabindu Upanishad 3)

Likewise, all yoga exercises are like carts on the road of yoga, being of crucial service to the practitioner in order to support a cleansing of tensions, unconsciousness or addictions. The more we realize the perspective of yoga, the more we have to learn to let go of the dependence on a practice. We may be grateful for having discovered the treasure of yoga practice, and yet we have to learn to stand on our own feet. Finally, we have to park our regular practice like the cart at the end of a road.

Exercise

It is not relevant what kind of practice you have. The basic principles of abhyasa and vairagya as mentioned so splendidly by Patañjali in the Yoga Sutras apply for physical exercises, breathing exercises, meditation as well as for all other forms of yoga practice. For our philosophical reflections abhyasa and vairagya play an important role as guidelines in order to inquire whether we are on the right path.

First, ask yourself to what extent you can manage to realize abhyasa, the moment of action, effort and concentration in your practice.

- *Do you always manage to muster up sufficient energy in order to practice regularly?*
- *What about your comfort zones? Can you always manage to overcome your weaker self to be active, to actually begin your practice and to carry through?*

In the next step ask yourself to what extent you are able to realize vairagya, the moment of non-attachment and relaxation.

- *Can you manage to relax and let go in your practice?*
- *Are you able to engage in your practice, to surrender to the practice and to let the practice happen?*
- *Can you practice without a sense of achievement and finally practice without wanting?*

In the beginning, abhyasa is primarily of importance in order to become active, to start with the practice and to carry it through. Then it is also important to cultivate vairagya: detachment from doing and effort. Yoga only truly becomes yoga once we can manage both moments of practice and non-attachment, and the magic way to achieve this is 'repetition'. Yoga is like brushing your teeth. It only helps a little if not done regularly. The regular repetition of yoga practice points towards a royal path, namely to reach deeper into mindfulness and to create focused ease. This way, one can increasingly learn to experience a force of lightness and less so one of doing. The union of abhyasa and vairagya, of active and passive, which is so hard to grasp in the beginning, now turns into a concrete experience.

9

The Philosophy of *Asanas*

Today's most popular type of yoga is *hatha yoga*. *Hatha yoga* begins with the physical practice of *asana*. But what is the exact meaning of the Sanskrit term *asana* that refers to the physical exercises? The literal translation of *asana* is seat or seated posture, but one is rarely sitting when practicing *asanas*. The literal meaning refers back to the historic origin of the exercise and can only be understood by going back in time in the history of yoga.

The practice of yoga did not begin with today's popular physical exercises of *hatha yoga*. When yoga was discovered perhaps around the 6th or 7th century BC, meditation emerged as the most important practice. However, for meditation it was initially crucial to be able to sit well. Likewise, in the oldest texts of yoga, the *Upanishads*, the right way of sitting as preparatory exercise for meditation was emphasized.

Later along the line, when *Patañjali* composed his Eightfold Path of Yoga, he also emphasized the practice of sitting rightly for meditation. He integrated the practice of sitting as the third limb of the eight limbs of yoga and called it *asana*, that is seat or seated posture. In the *Yoga Sutras* you can find a popular short definition of *asana*:

> *Sthira sukham asanam – The seated posture should be steady and comfortable.*
> *(Yoga Sutras by Patañjali 2.46)*

Patañjali does not describe a certain position of the legs or the arms and neither does it describe whether to have a straight spine or not. He only mentions two rather general principles on sitting, and these two principles seem to be contradictory at a first glance. Is it possible to hold a steady and stable seated posture and yet be comfortable and relaxed at the same time? Is a steady sitting posture not one at the expense of a comfortable one? Or vice versa, does not a comfortable seat usually lead to a posture that is less stable?

What is meant by 'steady' and 'stable' becomes more distinct once we compare the definition of the right sitting posture with *Patañjali's* previously mentioned yoga principles of *abhyasa* and *vairagya*. *Patañjali* called the first principle *abhyasa*, which means practice. In yoga it is important to be active and to make an effort in order to achieve firmness and stability. Through practicing *abhyasa* it becomes feasible to achieve a steady and stable seat, but for yoga the second principle *vairagya*, non-attachment, is essential, too. Only when we let go and relax, our seated posture becomes comfortable. The *asana* of yogic sitting realizes both principles at the same time. In the beginning the firmness when sitting can be mustered through effort. A regular practice supports mobility and flexibility of the body, so that it becomes possible to apply less effort in a seated posture, and to realize comfortable and relaxed stability in sitting. One can sit in firm stability and is entirely effortless at the same time. This pleasant stability emerges from releasing all tensions and from opening up for the inner center. The force of a good sitting posture results from the lightness of resting in one's Self. This is not about an outer, but an inner stability coming from the force of infinity. Hence, for *Patañjali asana* is so much more than simply preparation for meditation as stated in the *Upanishads*. From now on *asana* as the practice of sitting appears to be upgraded to a full-fledged yogic exercise.

Hatha yoga, which emerged later from the 10th century AD onwards, built upon these principles of the classical yoga of *Patañjali* and has developed them further. Meditation was also important for the *hatha* yogis, but they discovered the very particular role of the body for a holistic growth of man. After almost 2000 years when the center of a yogic practice had been the development of mind, it now became clear that the body also had to be integrated into this developmental process. The *hatha* yogis came up with physical exercises that no one had ever seen before in the history of yoga. They placed these exercises at the beginning of their yogic practice and called them *asana*, thus referring to the third limb of *Patañjali's* eight limbs of the *Yoga Sutras*. They had good reason for doing so. Even though these *asanas* had little in common with sitting, the seated postures became a basis for furthering a physical practice. Hence, from seated postures emerged variations of twisted postures, inversions, standing postures and postures in lying down. Countless variations of these classical *asanas*, but also various entirely new physical postures, have emerged since, not to mention the more dynamic physical exercises, which are continuously gaining in popularity.

Furthermore, *hatha yoga* managed to build beautifully upon the philosophy of *asana*. The physical exercises of *hatha yoga* are also supposed to be steady and yet comfortable. They demand the activity and effort of practice, but at the same time they are about letting go and being carried through the practice. The physical exercises show us how it is possible to reach into the infinity of the inner center with the body and to even live from this force of inner lightness. Thus, *hatha yoga* has managed to incorporate the principles of *Patañjali* and apply them practically on a physical level.

When *hatha yoga* refers to *asana* as physical practice it means everything that has already been said about *asana* in the sense of sitting rightly, and even more. Through *asana* as physical practice it becomes possible to directly target not only mental but also physical blockages. It becomes possible to cleanse the body of tensions and unconsciousness in a very specific manner in order to train awareness and inner vitality of mind and body. The yogic pathway has now expanded to a holistic process of growth, beginning at a very basic level, but with the potential to lead man to the loftiest heights.

In this way, the traditional texts refer to strengthening, relaxation and stillness of the body in the beginning of the practice. Further, they refer to enhanced digestion and improved physical health, but also to therapy for certain physical or mental illnesses. Yet, the impact of *asana* goes much further. Dissolving blockages is a requirement for an inner flow of energy. This is the so-called *pranic* energy, an inner energy that is closely related to the vitality of breath. Once *prana* is flowing, it in turn is a requirement to awaken an even deeper hidden, divine energy called *kundalini*. *Kundalini* can rise up from the pelvic floor and leads to the experience of *samadhi*, inner union, the awakening of our true, divine Self as enlightenment of body and mind.

With the prospect of experiences of *samadhi*, *hatha yoga* again builds on *Patañjali*. The *asanas* as physical exercises of *hatha yoga* are a point of entry to practicing yoga. Through *asanas* physical health can be improved and also certain illnesses can be treated. Yet, the perspective of the physical practice itself goes beyond these first effects. *Asanas* prepare the body for the experience of inner union and for the experience of the divine Self, which since the initial discovery of yoga have been found to be the true perspective of yoga.

Exercise

Looking at the history of yoga, we can distinguish between three areas as for the philosophy of asana: First, the philosophy resulting from the old Upanishads; second, the one resulting from the classical Yoga Sutras by Patañjali; and third, the one of hatha yoga. For today's yoga practice we can learn a lot from all three areas.

1. The experience of the importance of sitting rightly as mentioned in the Upanishads:

The old Upanishads know asana as the practice of sitting rightly as preparation for meditation. When our limbs and back hurt from sitting, meditation becomes very challenging. Accordingly, one would suggest to practice sitting before meditation.

2. The philosophy of asana according to classical-philosophical yoga by Patañjali:

The classical Yoga Sutras provide important guidelines for good sitting. These guidelines can be applied to seated meditation as well as to any other physical exercise. Patañjali describes a good asana as one that is 'steady' and 'comfortable'.

Examine the steadiness of both your seated posture as well as your entire physical practice:

- *What kind of steadiness do you experience? Is it more active or does it come without any effort?*
- *Do you have to summon up a lot of strength or does the steadiness come by itself without any additional doing?*

In asana, yogic stability emerges when firmness is comfortable at the same time. Stability comes automatically once we apply less effort and once the force of lightness begins to carry the practice. In your practice now search for experiences, where steadiness and comfort appear at the same time and where you can feel a force of lightness.

- *Apply the two principles of firmness and letting go as the two basic motives to further your future yoga practice.*

3. The development of asana as physical practice in hatha yoga:
Only hatha yoga has developed asana to a full physical practice. In hatha yoga the yogic pathway begins with concrete physical exercises and bodily experiences.

- *Have you ever experienced in your asana practice how tense muscles have begun to loosen, and awareness for your body has increased?*
- *Have you felt concrete effects from your practice such as better health or fewer illnesses?*

The body, however, also functions as a vehicle for the highest enlightenment. As for hatha yoga, to grow in yoga means to open up for deeper experiential realms, which lie beyond any physical levels.

- *How far have you managed to penetrate into the realms of energetic experiences, which are referred to as prana or kundalini in Sanskrit?*
- *Have you experienced being carried by an inner force, which you did not 'make', but which carried you and is described as a 'divine' energy in Hatha Yoga?*

Even though you may not be able to fully grasp the impact of these last questions, yet it still is important to be aware to what extent a philosophical dimension in your asana practice is relevant.

10

The Philosophy of *Pranayama*

Once one has progressed further into the practice of *asanas*, the practice can be expanded with breathing exercises. The practice of breathing is one of the oldest forms of yoga practice. Already at the time of the *Upanishads* it was understood that breath and mind have a reciprocal effect on each other. It was observed that mental states of unrest such as rage, anger or excitement would lead to a restless and fierce breath, whereas a balanced mind is accompanied by calm breathing. The breathing exercises deploy this interconnection of mind and breath in order to affect mind, thought and emotions in return. Thus, the breathing exercises are to be understood as *pranayama*, i.e. regulation of the breath. They help to control the breath, to slow and calm it down in order to create a balancing effect on emotions, thoughts and mind.

While in the very beginning of the history of yoga, at the time of the *Upanishads*, the basic coherence between mind and breath was recognized and this aspect was utilized, the classical yoga of the *Yoga Sutras* of *Patañjali* took it a step further. *Patañjali* arranged specific breathing exercises and included them as the fourth limb into his Eightfold Path of Yoga. Once a good seated posture was achieved, next the practitioner was to attend to *pranayama*.

So, what is pranayama according to *Patañjali*? Through his analysis we can learn a lot about the inner structure of this practice of yoga. According to *Patañjali* breathing consists of three constantly recurring stages: inhaling, exhaling and the times of breathing pauses in between. It is vital to slow down and expand this general course of the breath through *pranayama*. One can create an acuteness in breathing, which in turn leads to subtler activities of the mind. When *Patañjali* describes his objective of the breathing practice, what he actually means is difficult to grasp. *Patañjali* now refers to a fourth stage of breath, which reaches beyond the three general breathing stages; but what could be meant by this fourth stage of breath besides inhaling, exhaling and the pauses in between? *Patañjali* explains that this fourth stage reaches beyond any inner or outer objects, beyond anything that can be seen externally or be imagined internally. Inhaling, exhaling and breath retention happen in a realm of outer objects. They are 'doable' and can be observed from the outside. It is not the aim to transfer this outer breathing to an internal realm, a realm of thought objects, and to just imagine breathing. The path to the fourth dimension of breath changes the entire breathing fundamentally. Whilst the first three stages of inhaling, exhaling and breath retention are doable, the fourth stage eludes anything that is doable. The fourth stage of breathing comes into existence once we begin to do less while breathing. Consequently, breathing reaches a fundamentally new quality. What is meant is to advance from a form of breathing that is done to one that rests in itself. The fourth form of breathing happens when we 'continuously do less' and in this way 'continuously receive more'.

When the breath rests in itself, so the mind also rests. Likewise, what we express in today's language with 'receiving more' refers not only to the breath, but also to thoughts and emotions. In this fourth stage of breathing the sheath of unconsciousness disappears, which had previously covered up inner enlightenment. Through calming down the breath comes a calming of mental activities. Tensions, addictions or emotional ties are like a mantle that covers our true inner Self, our inner enlightenment. Thus, 'the Fourth' does not mean an additional stage of breathing, but it is an opening for a life carried by inner stillness, breathing from the clarity of a calm mind resting in the Self.

The manifold breathing exercises of yoga ranging from alternate nostril breathing to complex *pranayama* only emerged later in *hatha yoga*. Moreover, the *hatha* yogis developed a discrete philosophy of *pranayama*. In contrast to *Patañjali* the *hatha* yogis did not differentiate between three, but four visible stages of breathing: inhalation, exhalation, breath retention after inhaling and breath retention after exhaling. Of all stages, breath retention is of crucial significance. When pausing the breath, there is stillness, and since the discovery of *pranayama* calming the breath has become central to yoga. Yet, it is not enough to simply pause the breath, although there are reports that some yogis have gained great fame for being able to hold their breath for a long time. It has continuously been emphasized that deliberately pausing the breath or suppressing breathing activities is not considered *pranayama* in its original sense.

Now it becomes obvious that one can distinguish between different stages with regard to the breathing process. However, that which constitutes the inner core of the breathing exercises of yoga always stays the same. *Patañjali* referred to the fourth stage of breathing, the kind of breathing that is 'not doable', in order to shed light on the breath from the purity of a mind resting in the Self. In order to express the same phenomenon, *hatha yoga* differentiates between deliberate breath retention and an unintentional stillness of breath, which is what *pranayama* eventually comes down to.

Initially, breathing exercises must be carried out deliberately like all other exercises, and thus they begin with feasible accomplishments of certain breathing techniques. In the beginning of the practice the breath can be retained in the pauses between inhalation and exhalation, or vice versa between exhalation and inhalation. The real progress in this exercise does not lie in the prolongation of such pauses. This would only elongate a deliberate pause in breathing. This is not what *pranayama* is about. The unintentional stillness of breath comes spontaneously and happens once the breathing cycle becomes more focused, more tranquil and more subtle. In the course of the exercise breathing composes itself through 'not doing', so that breath and likewise mental activities begin to rest. The 'fourth stage' of breathing according to *Patañjali* and the 'unintentional' stage of breath retention of *hatha yoga* seem to point to the same perspective of yogic breathing.

More so, for *hatha yoga* it is important to not only focus on the mental realm, but also on the body. Not only tensions, addictions or emotional attachments of mind and soul need to be dissolved when mind and breath come to rest in this manner. The focus must also be directed on tightness and blockages in the body. In very concrete images the texts of *hatha yoga* refer to a 'cleansing' of the channels running through the body, so that energy can flow. *Hatha yoga* draws on images which can easily be misunderstood. When energy channels in the body are blocked these are by no means tangible debris and impurities. When *hatha yoga* speaks of energy, it is neither physical, nor thermic, and under no circumstances electrical energy. Here, energy is not to flow through the channels like power in a supply line.

All the images of *hatha yoga* are concrete expressions of the subtlest experiences. Impurities in the channels point towards tensions and blockages in the physical body or even to unconsciousness and dullness or a lack of inner vitality and vigor. If *pranayama* is to foster inner catharsis, this cleansing means the dissolution of such tensions and the growth of awareness. When less is 'done', the more the practitioner experiences an energy, which does not only carry the mind and the psyche, but also the physical body. *Hatha* yogis call this energy *prana*, and they consider this not only to be the breath but the experience of the primal energy of life force per se. Once the breath can rest in itself and all tensions in body and mind have dissolved, the pre-requirements are established for the divine energy, *prana*, to flow and to pervade body and mind.

According to the texts of *hatha yoga*, the flow of *prana* can indeed lead to sound health, a beautiful body and even a long life. However, for the yogic process the inner effect is vital. The body becomes permeable and vibrant. The foundation is laid to penetrate further into the spiritual depth of human existence. Thus, the philosophy of *pranayama* is a process of revitalization and awakening from the external towards the internal, from the tangible towards the intangible body by means of various stages culminating in the final experience of the true, divine Self as the spiritual depth of humanity.

Exercise

The philosophy of pranayama has taken place in three developmental stages. First, in the Upanishads the basic principle of breathing was discovered. Then, for the first time Patañjali was able to analyze and reveal the path of breathing practice. Hatha yoga holds account for the development of a multitude of concrete breathing exercises as a physical and energetic practice. These three developmental stages will be brought into concrete awareness in the following exercise for reflection.

1. The fundamental experience of the breathing practice according to the Upanishads:

Try to recall when you last were enraged, angry or furious. In what way did you breathe then? Now recall a situation of calmness and contentment. You may discover that an unsettled mind leads to uneasy breathing, just like balanced mental states are in line with calm breathing. Conversely, the breathing exercises of pranayama try to affect emotions and thought through breath.

- *Observe how in the process of having a more composed breath in your pranayama practice the fluctuations and ties in your mental and emotional realm begin to untangle.*
- *Take this observation into your everyday life. In a situation of anxiety or stress try to breathe in a calm and relaxed manner and observe how this will impact your mental state and yield an inner stability.*

2. The philosophy of pranayama in the classical-philosophical yoga of Patañjali:

An initial systematic practice of pranayama was developed in the Yoga Sutras. Practice according to Patañjali and observe the three stages of breathing: inhalation, exhalation and breathing pauses in between. Bring to mind that all three stages are 'doable', i.e. you can influence them deliberately. You can decide to inhale and exhale faster or slower and within certain limits also determine the length of your breathing pauses. After having practiced this over a long period of time, observe how this impacts your breath. Your breathing may alter to what Patañjali referred to as "the fourth" stage of breathing. The sheath of tensions, addictions and emotional urges begins to dissolve and inner enlightenment can arise.

3. The physical/energetic dimension of pranayama in hatha yoga:

Hatha yoga brought about the various breathing techniques as we know them today. If you have already come across forms of pranayama in hatha yoga pay particular attention to the breathing pauses. You may notice that in the beginning of your pranayama practice you will deliberately determine the length of your breath retention. So, in this case observe how the pausing changes after you have practiced pranayama for a long time and over a longer period of time. Perhaps you will observe that your breath ensues to be calmer and almost happens by itself. Also observe how this intuitive stillness in breathing is accompanied with mental calmness.

Observe how pranayama can support the cleansing process in your body of tensions and unconsciousness, so that you can increasingly experience being carried by a force that is called prana in hatha yoga.

11

The Philosophy of Meditation

Meditation was developed very early nearly 3000 years ago at the time of the *Upanishads*, when the first yogis went on a search to open man up for the experience of the true Self. Initially, practicing yoga meant to meditate. In a popular analogy meditation was compared to making fire. Matches or modern lighters were unheard of at this time in ancient India. Fire was made with firewood. A small spindle stick was drilled into a bigger piece of wood to spark the fire. In this analogy from the *Upanishads*, the bigger piece of wood at the bottom resembles the body of the meditator and the spindle stick a *mantra*, i.e. a meditative word or phrase. The drilling of the spindle stick represents the continuous recitation of this *mantra*. In today's yoga meditation various meditation words or phrases are being used. In the past only one *mantra* was known, which until today is still considered the most important *mantra* of India: OM. Just like the spindle stick must be drilled over a long period of time, so a *mantra* must be recited over and over, first aloud, then more quietly and finally as a mental impulse only. Thoughts stop roaming about. The scattered awareness becomes concentrated and is directed inside. Finally, one becomes focused and calm.

Today, few have experienced using a spindle stick to spark a fire. Hence, it is easy to see that without much practice one may drill the stick, but not succeed immediately to spark a fire. Likewise, it is possible to meditate and recite a *mantra* over and over, and yet nothing will happen. Only after a long and enduring time of practice when the stick begins to drill more easily, almost automatically, something will happen, which goes beyond the imagination of the layman. Two pieces of wood can spark a fire! And likewise, constantly repeating a *mantra* prepares and fosters what seems to be impossible in meditation. By constantly repeating a *mantra* not only the concentration of the practitioner enhances, but also serenity and inner peace improve. Through this detachment a transparency of mind can arise from where the primal experience of yoga can be ignited just like fire. Intuitive awareness awakens. A breakthrough to the experience of the inner, divine center becomes feasible. This is a spark of clarity, a spark of enlightenment. The divine Self of the human begins to break open. As this picture reveals, meditation is actually a way of creating fire, but it is important here to be careful not to get burnt.

Since the *Upanishads* meditation had constituted the center of yoga practice. When centuries later *Patañjali* systemized the yoga practice in his *Yoga Sutras* in the Eightfold Path of Yoga he introduced the philosophical analysis of meditation for the first time, which became the centerpiece of his text. According to *Patañjali* meditation consists of three moments. These are the last three limbs of the Eightfold Path. Firstly, meditation begins with *dharana*, concentration. Any form of meditation has its beginning in the focus on an object. Such an object can be the *mantra* OM for example. The activities of the mind, which in everyday consciousness focus fleetingly on one thing or another, are now directed on solely one object.

To be concentrating does not necessarily mean to be meditating yet. Secondly, it is important to add *dhyana*. Through *dhyana* meditation actually becomes meditation. *Dhyana* is the practice of non-attachment, letting go and surrender. Concentration becomes looser, but not in a way that the mind begins to drift and wander off to the next object. On the contrary, meditation is about a focused detachment, a more subtle concentration. *Dharana* and *dhyana*, concentration and non-attachment, belong together and are the two sides of the meditation process.

In a profound transformational process tensions, addictions and emotional ties begin to dissolve, so that an inner clarity can emerge in which the experience of inner union unfolds. In Sanskrit this is called *samadhi*, the third moment of meditation.

In his philosophical analysis *Patañjali* summarizes in one term what had been expressed in the image of sparking a fire from firewood in the *Upanishads*, but *Patañjali* took it one step further. According to him all other exercises of yoga, which had appeared in the meantime, have an inner essence of meditation. Sitting can become meditation if performed in meditative stability and repose. Breathing exercises can be considered meditation when performed in meditative awareness. Even when a yogi acts in the hubbub of worldly life or when he withdraws all senses from worldly life and continuously internalizes, that practicing is always about an opening for the inner center; this is meditation. Sitting practice, breathing, the withdrawal of the senses from worldly life and even engaging in everyday life – all these are exercises of the Eightfold Path of Yoga and can have meditation as their inner essence. Yoga is meditation or vice versa; only once an exercise is a practice of meditation it becomes yoga. Only when the practitioner is able to realize both moments, *dharana* and *dhyana*, when physical as well as breathing exercises together result in focus and repose, we can speak of yoga. Then and only then does the opportunity to tap into *samadhi* as the third moment, the force of the true Self, the experience of a union with the inner essence, become feasible.

Patañjali laid the foundation for the philosophy of meditation on which all following developments of yoga up to the present day are built. *Hatha yoga* in particular does not only support the development of meditation in correspondence with the physical practice, the *asanas* or the various breathing meditations, *pranayama*. Moreover, besides the *mantra* OM various other *mantras* are being practiced. The root *mantras lam, vam, ram, yam* and *ham* are for example some of the most popular. When chanted aloud in the beginning and later on recited silently, these *mantras* support an increasingly subtle mental attentiveness for vibrations resonating from the inner center without any audible sound.

Meditation on spatial objects, especially on concentration points within the body, is typical for *hatha yoga*. Such a focus point could be the point between the eyebrows or different energy centers along the spine. Moreover, meditation on *mandalas* has emerged, which is becoming increasingly popular today. These meditations begin with a focus on spatial images or objects in order to subtly direct the mind inwards and open it up for the experience of the inner light, which lies beyond any objective images. Especially through the developments of *Hatha Yoga* there are numerous meditation techniques that are available today and that are to be utilized.

Exercise

In order to understand what meditation is, it seems helpful to differentiate between two types of meditation. Meditation in its original sense is a mental practice on the one hand, and meditation in a broader sense points towards meditation as the essence of any yoga exercise on the other hand. Meditation in its original sense marks the beginning of the history of yoga and yoga practice. The first yoga exercise as referred to in the Upanishads is meditation as a practice of the mind. In the center of this meditation stood the mantra OM.

According to the Yoga Sutras of Patañjali the meaning of meditation was broadened. Besides meditation as the practice of the mind, now meditation in its wider sense was revealed as the essence of any yoga exercise. What turns yoga into yoga is referred to as meditation. Correspondingly, the physical practice that was introduced later on in hatha yoga can be considered a form of meditation with the body as the object of focus.

In the following exercise you can train your awareness for meditation as the inner essence of your practice.

- *The first moment of meditation as referred to by Patañjali is dharana, the focused concentration on an object. In your yoga practice bring to mind this moment of dharana. Where is your focus when you are practicing yoga? Is it perhaps on the body, the breath, the senses, a mantra, a mandala, a particular action or some sort of object?*
- *The second moment of meditation is dhyana, that is letting go, repose or detachment. Only by applying dhyana, meditation becomes meditation. Again observe your yoga practice and notice how your practice may change over time. How, when you practice consistently, does your concentration change? Notice how you begin to do less, how repose and lightness begin to*

emerge and how your practice begins to flow.

- *Dhyana is the prerequisite for samadhi, the experience of union. Feel how in your practice in the lightness of letting go a new force can emerge, which is not your 'doing'. Integrate the idea of 'doing less' into your practice, which eventually will lead to a 'receiving more'. This way you can open up for the experience of union, for a life from the innermost center of your being as the greatest perspective of all yoga practice.*

12

Karma Yoga – Yoga of Action

For many centuries, long before the physical practice of *hatha yoga* was established, the yogis had practiced through withdrawal into meditation. Yoga was considered to be a retreat from the hustle and bustle of everyday life to a place of stillness in order to turn inwards. In this way, yoga was a path that only few could take. It was only for those who had the opportunity to withdraw and live a life of meditation. Already *Patañjali* pointed out that the way inside was crucial for yoga, but overall it was more than a withdrawal from the world. Eventually, the way inside leads to new, more mindful engagement amidst the world.

Karma yoga shows that yoga cannot only be lived in the midst of the world, but that action itself can turn into a practice. The Sanskrit term *karma* means 'action'. Consequently, *karma yoga* literally means 'the yoga of action'. A *karma* yogi does not practice through withdrawal into the stillness of meditation; neither is his object of practice a mantra that turns his mind inwards. *Karma yoga* is practicing with action itself as the object.

The oldest and most important text on *karma yoga* is the *Bhagavadgita*, which appeared roughly 2000 years ago. Also, in various more recent scriptures the topic of *karma yoga* was addressed, but none of these interpretations managed to reach the same conceptual depths of the *Bhagavadgita*. The *Bhagavadgita* asks: "If yoga is an internal process of transformation, why should this inner process of transformation only be possible by withdrawing into meditation?" If meditation uses a *mantra* for practice and *pranayama* uses the breath, why should it not be possible to practice yoga through action and hence make yoga available for much wider levels of the population? *Karma yoga*, the yoga of action in everyday life, was born.

But how does *karma yoga* work? Practicing *karma yoga* means to act in the midst of everyday life without being attached to 'the fruits of the actions'. What are 'the fruits of the actions'? These are the effects of our actions. There are positive 'fruits' or effects of actions, such as recognition, rewards and success. Experience shows that actions can also bear 'foul fruits', such as criticism, punishment or failure. When we act in everyday life, we try to reap many of the positive 'fruits' and avoid the negative ones. Our actions are aligned to their results; we are constrained by them or as the *Bhagavadgita* says we are attached to the 'fruits', the effects of our actions. If we are attached to the fruits of our actions our mind is merely aiming at success and tries to avoid failure. The awareness for our Self, our true Self, is lost.

Karma yoga deals with this attachment to the fruits of our actions. Practicing *karma yoga* means to act in the midst of everyday life, like everyone else does, but with an entirely new mindset. First, the exercise is to become aware of one's own attachments to certain fruits, such as attachments to recognition, rewards or success. It is important to identify these attachments in order to be able to gradually let go of them. The aim is to become less dependent on the results of one's actions such as success or failure. Once the dependence decreases the practitioner can experience calmness and stability from the inner center. When this stability intensifies, the dependences on the fruits of actions begin to dwindle. What makes yoga yoga and what characterizes all yogic pathways begins to happen. That process of inner transformation, the 'undoing' of the ties on worldly matters, begins to happen so that awareness for the inner center, the true Self, can emerge.

Karma yoga provides a practical pathway that can be exercised anywhere. The *Bhagavadgita* even depicts the most extreme situation to practice in, which is the situation of war. Whilst traditionally yoga is practiced through withdrawal from society to a place of silence and peace, now a place is described that could not be more contradictory: a battlefield shortly before the outbreak of the biggest battle ever described in Indian literature. If *karma yoga* can be practiced in such an extreme situation, consequently it can be practiced in any other conceivable situation.

The warrior is facing the great battle and knows that his victory will bring him the fruits of fame, honor and power, but also the painful death of his opponent. Not to fight would spare the opponent but would also leave the power to the opposing side. Victory and defeat, honor and disgrace, all these are the fruits of action. Practicing *karma yoga* here means to stop aligning one's actions to their fruit. Here, the warrior has to embed his mind to his true Self and to act independently of the fruits of his actions, victory or defeat. In directing the mind to the true Self of the present, the *karma* yogi does what is necessary in the very moment.

In today's *karma yoga* practice in certain yoga centers, smaller fruits are considered. *Karma yoga* is practiced when cooking in the kitchen, when cleaning toilets or when weeding a garden. The fruits of the actions then are the delicious food, clean toilets, a garden free of weeds or perhaps even praise for having done a good job. Yet, the principle is the same. Whether the fruits are victory or defeat in a battle or clean toilets, nevertheless *karma yoga* means to let go of the attachment to success or failure as the fruit of the action, and to reflect on our true purpose in life, that which really matters. What matters is the experience of abundance in every moment, from where awareness for what is necessary becomes clear. Through detachment from our inner ties of success or failure we are to cultivate a force and energy, which enables us to act from our inner center of the true Self.

Exercise

For the following exercise on karma yoga look for a place to practice within your everyday life. It is helpful to consider a situation where the success of your action has not eventuated yet, but perhaps you are to face a result quite soon. Such places of practice can be the kitchen, where you do your dishes, cleaning your house, weeding in the garden or standing in a queue in a supermarket. Practice karma yoga in three steps:

- *First, become aware of how you are attached to the fruits of your actions. Ask yourself why you are acting? Is it the cleanliness of the dishes, your house or your garden, or perhaps a materialistic reward on reaching the checkout, or recognition of your success? Notice how mind and body are divided. While your body is acting in the present, your mind is focused on the future fruits of action.*
- *Secondly, bring your mind back into the present away from the future success of your acting. Now, while you are doing your task, try not to consider the results of your actions any longer but become completely present. Take on the stance of an observer, who watches over you in full awareness in the here and now. Observe how you do your dishes, clean your house, do the gardening or queue in a line in a supermarket.*
- *As a third step, try to enjoy the very present moment in the here and now. Cultivate a 'presence without any expectations', a stability of inner calmness while you are acting, and practice awareness for what is necessary. Most likely this will emerge after having practiced karma yoga over a period of time.*

Once you are able to practice karma yoga in such easy situations, move on to a field of practice in which it is harder for you to loosen the attachment to the fruits of your actions and cultivate mindfulness in the present of the here and now.

IV. The Big Topics of Yoga

13

Yogic Experiences

In the beginning of our yoga practice we are usually quite satisfied if back pains begin to alleviate, we find better sleep at night or when the body becomes more flexible and agile. Some say that the true yogic experiences are extraordinary occurrences such as visions, certain states of bliss or 'out-of-body' experiences. Yet others describe certain states of immersion beyond time and space. The philosophical texts report of experiences of union with 'the Absolute', a conscious life from the center or the true Self. So, which of these manifold possibilities of experiences can be considered yogic? Is it only the *one*, or several or even all of them?

A great aid in order to assess yogic experiences is to divide them into four categories in a first instance. The first category contains experiences that have been affected externally. Usually these experiences are also the first to ensue when physical or mental ailments such as back pains, headaches or insomnia begin to cease. The breath becomes calmer and more subtle. The bodily functions become increasingly steady through the practice. What a fantastic beginning, but only a beginning. These first experiences are very important, but they only point to the surface of what is possible in yoga. Yoga is a very helpful technique at this level of treatment. The exercises constitute external stimuli, which in return lead to the desired positive effects. For example, a perfectly performed headstand is such an external stimulus. What is characteristic about such externally initiated exercises is that the experience usually ceases when stopping the practice. Most likely the return of back pains, headaches or insomnia will not take too long.

However, it is indeed possible to further develop one's yoga practice and enter a new dimension of yogic experiences. This is the second category of experiences. So far we have claimed that through more practice we will gain more, but in the second category this is inevitably not so any longer. Now these experiences arise when 'doing less'. This is a very specific 'doing less'. The practitioner does less in his practice and thus enables a transformational process of inner renewal. An entirely new force begins to carry, which is a force of lightness, of flow, an experience of inner stability and an inner state of being borne.

This process of transformation occasionally happens in states of disruption, where intense energies can be released quite suddenly. Spontaneous muscular convulsions are possible. The practitioner may be overwhelmed by feelings of bliss or light or sound appearances. Once the sheaths of consciousness begin to loosen progressively, some may have extraordinary experiences such as visions or out-of-body experiences. These experiences are also accessible beyond a yogic practice for people with special medial aptitudes, for people who a priori possess a special permeability for the so-called subtler dimensions of cognition and being. Such extraordinary experiences are not always benign. They bear the great risk of a new form of attachment when great yogis exhibit a show of such experiences, and competition ignites over the most spectacular skills. Extraordinary experiences can happen, but they do not have to. They are only some sort of by-product on the yogic pathway. What is crucial for this second category is the experience of progressively 'doing less' in order to be borne more. The experience of the second dimension is not practiced through a yogic technique, but is fostered through a regular yoga practice in order to almost emerge on its own without any additional doing.

Once the second category is achieved through 'doing less', which fosters a 'receiving more', so in the third category 'doing nothing' in order to 'receive everything' is the maxim. Accordingly, the *Hatha Yoga Pradipika*, one of the most important texts on *hatha yoga*, says:

> *As camphor transcends in fire and salt dissolves in water*
> *So mind dissolves when one with the true Self.*
> *(Hatha Yoga Pradipika 4.59)*

All doing ceases, and so does all thinking. All doing and thinking disappear like camphor in fire and salt in water; nothing is left. All there is is life, truthful life, life from the inner center. All attachments and tensions in body and mind but also thoughts and feelings, desires and beliefs have dissolved. While the motions of the mind begin to settle, the experience of inner stability emerges. Deep serenity manifests itself as well as the awareness for the true Being, for what we actually and originally are.

Various terms have emerged in order to describe this third dimension of yogic experience. What is meant is *samadhi*, which can be translated as 'union' or 'immersion' or *kaivalya*, 'absolute non-attachment', but just like camphor and salt disintegrate in fire or water, so these terms too begin to disintegrate. This dimension describes an experience which cannot be grasped through certain terminology. These yogic experiences constitute the essential, ineffable nature of yoga practice; and yet, the end on the yogic pathway has still not been reached.

So far, we have focused on the internal experiences of our yoga practice. The fourth category goes beyond practice. This fourth category has the potential to fundamentally change the life of the practitioner. It is the experience of 'union' or 'absolute non-attachment' in the midst of the turmoil of everyday life. For most of us it is easier to experience inner stability of yogic serenity through a withdrawal from a hectic life. As such, yogic exercises of withdrawal are part of a general practice. However, many texts and schools warn of stagnation in a retreated life from the world. The serenity of the practice deepens when lived in the midst of everyday life and when it remains vibrant there. The essence of this dimension is to permeate everyday life with a mind of original vitality.

Even though we have categorized yoga experiences in four consecutive dimensions, it is not necessary to align ourselves to one of these, in order to understand where we are on our own yogic journey. It is not possible to reduce a human being to one single place on his yogic journey. For example, in certain areas the practitioner may have opened up for deep yogic experiences while in other areas of their life certain ties or attachments may have not dissolved yet. The above structure of yogic experiences is too simplistic to meet the complexity of the yogic journey. Just like camphor and salt disintegrate in fire and water, structure and categories dissolve once yoga turns into a concrete experience. Yet, these categories can be seen as a useful map of yogic experiences in order to give direction and provide hints on what to look for.

Exercise

The above four categories can help you to better understand your own yogic experiences. For the following exercise have a pen and paper at hand. First, bring to mind what kind of yogic experiences you have had so far and write down keywords with regard to these experiences. In a second step, try to classify your yogic experiences according to the four categories:

- *Which experiences belong to the first category of the externally-technically motivated practice of yogic experiences?*
- *Which of your experiences belong to the second category of 'doing less' and 'receiving more' in return, where you experience a flow, a force of lightness or even by-products such as extraordinary experiences?*
- *Which of your experiences fit in the third category, where all thinking and all doing dissolve like salt in water, where we are in deep serenity, not doing anything, and at the same time experiencing our true being?*
- *To what extent has the fourth dimension opened up for you; where it is possible to remain in deep serenity, not in reclusiveness, but in the midst of the hustle and bustle of everyday life?*

Please bear in mind that such categories can be helpful. However, the yogic pathway is not one of categories but a concrete, experiential practice, which ultimately reaches far beyond all our attempts to create structures and definitions.

14

Master and *Guru*

Is it necessary to study with a master of yoga? The possibilities to learn yoga today are widely available. Numerous books, DVDs and CDs make it possible to practice at home without a teacher. Many institutions offer yoga courses. If you look at the Indian tradition the personal yoga lessons were largely embodied by the close relationship between the master, called *guru*, and his student. For the time of study, the master would take the students he had adopted into his *ashram*, that is his yoga center, or even into his family. Likewise, the close relationship between master and student became the central pillar of the teachings of yoga. For a long time study texts and practical assignments were delivered only orally. Various traditions emerged, through which yoga was transmitted from master to student and from this student to the next student, not only for generations, but for centuries without the existence of any written evidence.

In ancient India the necessity of a master did not need to be emphasized. If you wanted to learn yoga, the only way to do so was to study with a master of yoga. Further, the master and *guru* fulfilled an important role in providing the student with a foothold and security. In the turmoil of everyday life the student could rely on his master with certainty to find the truth of yoga with him. The awareness of being taught by a master of a long-standing tradition, who had been in touch with grand masters of the past, would give the student assurance of being on the right path. A master would grant the seeker confidence of being well and properly guided on the path of yoga.

This close student-teacher-relationship describes the teaching practices of ancient India, but a lot has changed in India today.

Especially in Western countries the term *guru*, a master of yoga, has got a mostly negative connotation. Moreover, in Western cultures the strict subjugation to a master does not correspond with the ideal of a modern, responsible human, who wants to determine his own life. In the pluralism of the present the belief that there is only one single path of truth has increasingly dwindled away. Because nowadays yoga can be studied independently of any historic lineage it is not necessary to commit to one single yoga tradition. Often even techniques off the yogic path, ranging from Buddhist meditation to progressive muscular relaxation, are being integrated into one's own yoga practice. The competence of the master and *guru*, who used to determine what the student had to learn, has shifted to a self-determined student, who himself chooses from today's diverse range of yoga what meets his personal needs best. The foothold that the focus on the one master and the one true tradition used to provide is replaced by the foothold of the modern human being himself, who is knowingly able to determine his own life.

But what now is the better way to learn yoga? Does it comply more with yoga to surrender to a *guru* or to one tradition in order to learn genuine yoga from a genuine master? Or is it better to follow the ideal of the responsible human being, who is able to take control over his own life, who picks what is good from various masters and leaves the bad aside? The master or ourselves, who is to decide?

The answer according to yoga is: neither master nor ourselves. Surely, a yoga teacher is important. Learning from books alone is difficult and can also be dangerous. It is the teacher in particular who can point out false postures or false developments, and who provides important assistance. However, a good yoga practice also lives from the own initiative of the practitioner himself and from a critical search for one's own pathway, the one that is good and right for oneself. For some the relationship with a teacher or even master is important in order to gain a foothold on the path of yoga and to gain valuable personalized direction. For others it is better to be self-determined and to practice yoga independently. Master and independence do not constitute alternatives. They are means for something higher altogether, namely that which concerns yoga in its actual and original sense.

Already some 2000 years ago, *Patañjali* the author of the *Yoga Sutras* has pointed towards the path to the *guru* of all *gurus*, towards the master of all masters. This is the master within us, and to awaken this master should be the endeavor of all external masters of yoga. This true master within us may not be confused with our everyday self, which continuously tries to take control over our life and tries to determine us. The true master lies deeply within us. It is our true Self that is to be experienced in the depths of our very own existence.

Since ancient times this *guru* of all *gurus* has been referred to by the Sanskrit term *antaryamin*, 'the inner guide'. Once consciousness has cleared and the practitioner has gained security, he then will no longer need an outer foothold of a master or an 'ego'. The student will then be guided from within, from his inner *guru* as a voice of his true Self. The essence of all yoga practice lies in the discovery of this true inner *guru*. This could be through a traditional master-student-relationship as well as through a responsible examination of the present.

According to an old image, the yogic pathway is compared to a passage through a gate. For some a master is this gate, through which the student has to go if he wants to reach his true Self. However, the risk here is that the student may not step through the gate, but will stop just in front of it in order to hold on to it or even to worship it. Clinging to a master provides a foothold and security, yet it may hinder growth on the yogic pathway, which the student himself needs to enable.

For the modern person the gate is not the master, but his own Self. The allegedly responsible student himself determines which path he wants to take and which not. "*I myself am the gate to* which *I* hold on to." Yet, here again it is important to progress and this means to find one's true Self. Surely, one will not succeed after one single yoga class. Thus, it seems helpful to hold on to a master or *guru* in order to find security, and only then continue on the path. Eventually, growing in yoga means to change oneself, to let go of any attachments to a master and likewise of the ego in order to awaken to what really serves, 'the inner guide' as the true master and *guru*.

Exercise

To be on the path of yoga can mean that we have found a gate which gives our lives direction. In the following exercise bring to mind where you are standing yourself in yoga. What is your gate in yoga?

- *Is it a teacher or even a master who will tell you how you can practice? Bring to mind how helpful it can be to have found such a teacher who can point you to the treasures of yoga.*
- *Or do you rather consider yourself a modern and responsible human being, who takes on the beneficial aspects of teachers and masters and leaves aside the rest? Bring to mind how helpful it can be to find a gate as a point of entry to yoga in yourself, and walk this path self-determinedly.*

According to the ancient metaphor of the yogic pathway as a passage through a gate, both ways mentioned enjoy equal rights. Both ways give us directions which our lives can take. Why should we not allow ourselves to hold on to a path that we have found and that gives us direction?

However, the deeper sense of yoga lies not in holding on, but in passing through a gate, so that we can grow and transform ourselves.

- *Ask yourself where you are standing on your passage through this gate. Are you more drawn to a master or to a self-determined life?*
- *Bring to mind that both a master and we ourselves are like gates. They are important as they point towards an entry, but they are also there to walk through.*

Give yourself time to reflect when it is important for you to hold on to something in order to not loose ground or to not topple over. Bear in mind that yoga also means to let go of a teacher or a master and also of the ego. Yoga means to move beyond any gates in order to become centered within and to awaken to 'your inner guide', the master of all masters.

15

Yoga and Religion

In most Western countries yoga is taught as a practice to maintain good health of body and mind. Many vehemently reject the idea that yoga has something to do with religion. However, a glimpse into the Indian tradition reveals that the oldest texts, the *Upanishads*, were worshiped as religious texts. The *Bhagavadgita*, one of the most important books of yoga, is referred to as 'the bible' of Hinduism, and as a matter of fact in India a prayer is usually spoken in the beginning of the yoga practice. Often a specific religious yoga is practiced, *bhakti yoga*, the yoga of religious devotion. So, how can the connection between yoga and religion be conceived? In order to answer this question substantially, first the phenomenon of religion needs to be clarified. What is religion? In fact, there are four central traits in any religion. With reference to these four traits, it can be revealed how yoga and religion can be seen as fundamentally different on the one hand and how on the other hand they are closely interrelated.

First, in any religion the belief in a god is prevalent. Some believe in god as a person opposite us. Others see in god an impersonal force or a rather abstract concept. Some believe god to be male, others female and yet others believe it to include both sexes or none at all, as the concept of god cannot be comprehended in this way. Monotheistic religions such as Judaism, Christianity and Islam believe in 'one' god. Asian religions such as Hinduism, Buddhism or Daoism know 'many' gods. In each case, there is a belief system about a force beyond human power, which this world is based on or from which the world is driven.

Does this mean that one has to believe in god or even in the Hindu gods when practicing yoga? Surely, yoga does not exclude religion. Hindus in India practice yoga just like Christians practice yoga passionately in the West. Consequently, a Hindu will most likely pray at the beginning of the practice, perhaps in order to ask for guidance in his practice from the gods. That does not make yoga a religion. You can but you do not need to pray or believe in god in order to practice yoga.

It can be noticed, however, that for religious people often the faith in god may change over time if they have been on the yogic journey for a while. Some, who used to believe themselves to be somewhere beyond on the religious journey, report that through the experiences in their yoga practice they have rediscovered the original meaning of religion. However, the belief or faith which these people rediscover is a new and transformed belief. Yoga means to walk an experiential path, and likewise for the religious person religion becomes an experiential journey. The belief in a god far away and beyond transforms into an experience of being borne by a larger more comprehensive dimension. The experience that what is crucial in our lives cannot be 'done' begins to manifest. Yogis experience that what is crucial in life is 'given' to us. Yoga leads the practitioner to his inner essence, the experience of one's very own existence, which is understood by religious people as the divine inherent nature of humanity. Admittedly, there is no need to interpret these experiences from a religious point of view or to link them to religion. However, a religious person would most likely do so and interpret the yogic experiences as experiences of divine truth, as the primal form of religious life.

However, religion is not only the faith in a god. A second trait that all religions have in common is the belief in religious teachings. In the teachings all religions deliver answers to the central questions of human existence. Accordingly, within religions doctrines of creation, reincarnation, life after death or of a last judgment have emerged. All these doctrines deal with the central questions: Where do I come from? Who am I? To where will I go? Yoga also has doctrines. Partly, some of these religious doctrines have been integrated into textbooks on yoga. However, all doctrines, religious teachings or others only constitute a beginning, a point of entry to the yogic pathway. You could also say that doctrines are like the surface, an outer sheath for the inner essence of yoga, for the actual meaning of yoga. Yoga wants so much more than can be grasped through religious teachings. In yoga the central questions on human existence are not answered through doctrines that one must believe in. Yoga is a path of change and transformation, through which we can experience directly where we have come from, who we are, and to where we will go. For some the religious teachings or certain doctrines may be of great importance in the beginning, but once the growth in yoga practice has lead to the experience of the inner fruits of yoga, they begin to appear as only an outer sheath, enclosing the inner fruit of direct vital experience.

Now we have reached the third trait of religion, the belief in commandments, which are to guide our worldly activities. As a matter of fact, many of the commandments of various religions are of a similar nature. Yet, others may be very different. What they all have in common is to determine what kind of actions are of good conduct and to prevent those that are considered bad conduct. Often religions hold out the prospect of some sort of reward for good conduct and punishment in case of any violations of the commandments. As such a Hindu yogi will pay respect to the commandments of Hinduism just like a Christian yogi will respect the commandments of Christianity. An Atheist yogi may observe his own rules and regulations or perhaps legal ones, such as only the traffic regulations. However, very often a code of conduct, which has its roots in Hinduism, has found its way into the Western yoga communities. These behavioral standards may range from vegetarianism to taking the shoes off before entering a yoga hall. Again, like the religious doctrines these behavioral standards are only a beginning, a point of entry or an outer sheath of what yoga truly is. Often commandments provide a foothold and security for those who have not penetrated yet to an inner discernment. For the religious practitioner the commandments of a specific religion begin to change with an increasing understanding of the deeper meaning of yoga. The practitioner will develop a deep internal understanding of what is good and bad conduct. Furthering one's yoga practice will lead to a growth of inner strength in order to realize what has been experienced as good and righteous from the depth of one's very own existence.

As the last of the four traits of religion the practice of rituals and that of cults must be mentioned. Religions find their ritual expression in sacrifice, worship or cult. The religious cult of worshiping the gods, which has its fixed place in India, can be seen as only the beginning and a point of entry of an outer sheath of yoga, as various Indian ashrams do not limit their practice to that of *asanas*. As soon as the divine is not only recognized in heaven, but also in the very inner nature of man, praying to the gods will change. Worship and cults themselves can become the practice for the religious practitioner. Worship becomes the pathway of the yogic practice, namely that of *bhakti yoga*, the yoga of religious devotion. In yoga, what initially is external sacrifice turns into a practice of inner devotion and of an inner surrender, which will open the practitioner for the divine experience. Likewise, verbally uttered prayers will lead to silence, and lastly to a listening and an awareness for what really carries in our lives.

Both are right when some people argue that yoga has nothing to do with religion while others emphasize that yoga opens one up for the inner life and the depths of religion. Yoga is a pathway of transformation, and of growth in inner depth and in the experience of our primordial life. In the Indian tradition this pathway is understood to be religious and at the same time nonreligious. Important religious texts of Hinduism such as the

Upanishads or the *Bhagavadgita* are testimonies of the religiously interpreted primordial experiences of yoga. On the contrary, the *Yoga Sutras* of *Patañjali* offer a yogic pathway independent of religion.

Whether the yogic pathway is understood to be a religious one or not is of no major importance. Ultimately, the various yogic pathways can be compared to an ascent up a rooftop, according to an analogy by the great Indian sage *Ramakrishna*. You can reach the rooftop via a stony staircase or via a wooden one. You can ascend up a bamboo ladder or use a rope. You can even climb up with the help of a bamboo pole or with your bare hands only. Just like there are various ways up to the rooftop, there are various nonreligious yogic pathways besides the religious one. What is crucial is to not remain on the ground floor of life and to live with dependences and in unconsciousness, but to walk a path of change and transformation, which will lead you to the top of the roof – where religious and nonreligious people can meet. Whether religious or not, it is crucial to accept as true that there is a roof on which to exploit one's full potential, to grow and to open up for the experience of what really carries in this life.

Exercise

For the following exercise imagine your life to be a room on the ground floor of a house, which has a staircase to the roof.

- *How is your room of life furnished? Is there any religious or spiritual decoration?*
- *Is the belief in a divine force important for you?*
- *Do religious teachings or doctrines provide a foothold and security for you?*
- *Do you believe in religious commandments?*
- *Do you have a religious practice such as prayer or rituals?*
- *Or is your room a nonreligious space? Perhaps you do not believe in a god and have a more worldly orientation?*
- *How is the room of your life designed?*

When you practice yoga and do so with endurance and surrender, your life will begin to change. To be on the path of yoga does not mean to go out and buy new furniture, nor to buy a new yoga mat or displays of Hindu gods for your practice space. For yoga it is not important how the room of our life is furnished, meaning whether we live in a religious or nonreligious way. For yoga it is important whether we have found the staircase up to the rooftop and also whether we have tried to ascend up to the next floor. Hence, it is important to walk the way of practice that will lead to change. Perhaps one day we will reach the rooftop. There we can awaken to our inner essence, which will connect us in the innermost way with everything alive, regardless of being a Hindu, a Buddhist, a Daoist, Jew, Muslim, Christian or Atheist, and regardless of whether we consider ourselves to be religious or nonreligious.

16

The Theories of *Karma* and Reincarnation

Parallel to the question of yoga and religion other questions, which are closely related to the origins of Hinduism, have been discussed in yogic circles. "Is yoga inevitably related to the theory of *karma*?" Or: "As a yogi does one have to believe in reincarnation?" Also sometimes *karma yoga*, the yoga of practice in daily life, and the theory of *karma* are being confused. As such there is a need to first clarify what the theory of *karma* actually is, and also what is reincarnation from a Hindu point of view?

In order to find conclusive answers it is important to go back to the origins of the teachings, to the *Upanishads*. These texts provide the oldest testimonies in which both theories were introduced in ancient India. First, to address the theory of *karma*: *Karma* is a term from Sanskrit, which can be translated literally as 'action'. Thus, the theory of *karma* means 'action theory' or 'the teachings of actions'. The theory of *karma* explains how the actions of humans work. It implies that every action has an according effect and that this effect will eventually fall back onto the person, who has acted himself, though the effect may not materialize immediately nor directly after the preceded action. What is important is that no effect of any action that has been carried out is ever lost. A good action will sooner or later result in a positive effect on the executer. Likewise, bad actions will necessarily result in bad effects on the executer. Consequently, everyone is free to choose whether to top up their *karma* account in a positive way or whether to collect bad *karma*.

This in turn means that bad fortune or the sufferings of someone are considered the present effect of poor past action. On the other hand, good fortune and everything positive are the effects of good past conduct. It is impossible to escape one's own *karma*, which are the effects of one's own actions. Thus, the teachings of *karma* have found a way to explain why some people are more fortunate than others. There is a guaranteed punishment for the offender, but also the reward for the one who does good. *Karma* affects a person like destiny that has been caused by himself and which he cannot escape. Good fortune and bad fortune of any human being are determined by his or her actions. Only if one works off his bad *karma*, and is prepared to surrender to his misfortune and sufferings or if one improves his *karma* through good conduct will it become possible to change the course of one's destiny.

Of course, the question of what are good and what are bad actions needs to be addressed. It may be the case that one person considers an action good while another person regards the same action as bad. In order to provide more clarity the sacred Hindu texts determine that good conduct complies with the Hindu caste system. By contrast, actions that offend the caste system will produce bad *karma*. For example, if a *Brahmin*, a member of the highest caste of priests, eats with a Hindu of a lower caste or eats meat, which is considered impure, he will produce bad *karma*, but if he respects the Hindu food code this means good *karma*.

Consequently, the theory of *karma* has a significant impact on Hindu society. Hinduism does not know a last judgment after death according to which a god rewards good deeds with access to a heavenly paradise and punishes bad deeds with condemnation in purgatory and hell. Neither does Hinduism need an image of a last judgment to induce their believers into observing the commandments and prohibitions. A Hindu believes in the theory of *karma*, according to which rewards and punishments will happen naturally and by themselves solely based on one's actions. Hence, a theory was created that would urge the Hindu believer to observe the commandments. The individual is included and held in the *karmic* belief of a cosmic order and thus is provided with a foothold and security in this transient and impermanent world.

The theory of *karma* can explain a lot, but two important questions remain open. What will happen with certain *karmic* effects that have not materialized yet when someone is about to die? And why do people who always do good sometimes experience misfortune, and vice versa, why are people with bad intentions sometimes lucky? Another theory, which emerged around the same time and which is mentioned for the first time in the *Upanishads*, can provide answers to these questions. This is the theory of reincarnation.

In the oldest of the *Upanishads* the question emerged, what would happen with living entities after death? This question emerged independent of the theory of *karma*. If it is assumed that humans enter a world beyond, after they have died the question remains, why does this world not fill up? The answer here is, that the souls go to another realm after death, but they will return to this world after a certain time. The belief in reincarnation was created. After birth a human grows into an adolescent, then into an adult, which is followed by old age and physical death. Death, however, is followed by a new birth, a new growth etc. Without being aware of it, man has been on this earth many times and will reincarnate again and again countless times.

At the same time, the belief in reincarnation delivers the answer to the two remaining questions of the theory of *karma*. The first problem of what would happen with the effects of past actions of someone who is about to pass away was solved. The effects are not lost. They form the cause for a new birth, a new life in which they can materialize. Moreover, the misfortune of a good person and the good fortune of a bad person can now be explained. Good and bad fortune are the effects of actions carried out in a previous life, which have only materialized now, in the present.

Now, what does all this mean for yoga? Most Indian yogis who teach yoga are of Hindu descent and thus believe in the teachings of *karma* and reincarnation. These teachings, however, are only marginally concerned with yoga in its original sense. Like all other teachings that have evolved around yoga, so these are equal to an outer sheath only. In order to penetrate to the essence of yoga, it can be useful to start with the outer sheath. Yet, it is important not to remain there, but to break through further and open up for the yogic pathway of experience.

As a result, the theories of *karma* and reincarnation are particularly relevant for Indian yoga, but they need a specific yogic interpretation. From a yogic point of view the theory of *karma* refers to unconscious actions and attachments in our everyday lives. It explains how unmindful actions work, and how man is tied to the effects of his actions. He is tied to these effects as long as he only observes the commandments because his unconscious actions are aimed at rewards that he may hope for, or because he may be afraid of punishment. Based on the theory of *karma* one tries to create good *karma*, i.e. good effects and avoid bad *karma* and bad effects. Consequently, often all our strivings are solely aimed at gathering more wealth and more recognition, satisfying desires or even being reborn into a better realm. In this striving for more one is continuously driven until death and even further into a new life. As man is forced to be reborn, he will always be driven in the eternal cycle of rebirths.

This is where yoga comes in. To be on the yogic pathway does not mean to observe Hindu dos and don'ts in order to create good *karma* and to be reborn into a higher realm. It is not about believing in *karma* and reincarnation, nor about following any other theories or beliefs. To be on the yogic pathway means to be able to recognize one's own unconsciousness as well as one's own inner ties and attachments, which the theories of *karma* and reincarnation try to express. Whether such ties and unconsciousness are linked to the theory of *karma* or that of reincarnation is of no importance for the yogi. To be on the yogic pathway means to let oneself in for a transformational process, which will enable a detachment from the ties of the constant striving for wealth and recognition in order to open up for the experience of inner freedom.

Exercise

First bring to mind how significant the teachings of karma and reincarnation are for you as an outer sheath of yoga:

- *To what extent are the teachings of karma, which explain the effects of good and bad actions, helpful for you?*
- *To what extent can you identify with the theory of reincarnation, which provides an explanation for life after death?*
- *Are there any other theories or teachings that are convincing for you in order to explain the effects of our actions and life after death? Which are these?*
- *Or are you someone who do not need to explain any of these questions with the help of doctrines or theories?*

Independently of how you have answered the above questions, as for the fruit of yoga it is important to walk the yogic pathway in its original sense and not to adhere to any theories. Being on this pathway is a matter of becoming aware of our ties and attachments in order to dissolve them. As a consequence the following questions need to be addressed:

- *Do you know of any actions that are aimed at producing beneficial effects or at avoiding negative ones? Bring to mind how these actions are tied to the desired effects and also how these ties can obscure the awareness of actions resulting from the inner center of the Self.*
- *In your life, how much are you concerned about past or future reincarnations? Contemplate to what extent such a concern can conceal the awareness for the here and now as the fruit of yoga.*

Finally, contemplate that in yoga all theories including those of karma and reincarnation only constitute an outer sheath. Yoga only becomes alive once one manages to penetrate from the outer sheath of the teachings to the inner fruit of experience.

17

The Philosophy of OM

Since the times of the *Upanishads* up to the present day highest importance has been ascribed to the *mantra* 'OM'. In fact, 'OM' is much more than a *mantra*, a meditation word. In order to emphasize its uniqueness a written character has been ascribed to 'OM', which expresses this one sound only and is used in no other word. 'OM' cannot be translated into other languages, because 'OM' stands beyond any language. It is the primal sound per se. In this sense 'OM' not only comprises the nature of all languages, but also all words that have ever been uttered in any existing languages. 'OM' is the sound which encompasses all other sounds. It even embraces the entire world. 'OM' is the universe. The meaning of 'OM' reaches even beyond that. 'OM' is the path to experience and to the true Self. 'OM' is the true Self. How can all this be explained?

To do so it is important to refer back to the roots of the philosophy of 'OM' as can be found in the *Upanishads*. Here 'OM' is split into its individual components, each of which can be interpreted by itself. Pronounced as a sound, initially 'OM' breaks down into two parts: First 'O' and then an 'M' can be heard: 'OOOOOOOOMMMMMMMMM'.

In a next step it is assumed that the sound 'O' was composed through the contraction of the two individual sounds 'A' and 'U'. 'AAAAAAUUUUUU' turns to 'OOOOOO'. When conversely 'O' is deconstructed into its original sounds 'A' and 'U' emerge. This way it becomes possible to differentiate between the three

---

Throughout this chapter, when referring to the sound 'A', it is pronounced as in 'calm'; and when referring to the sound 'U' it is pronounced as in 'mood'.

sounds of 'OM': 'A', 'U' and 'M'. In addition, it is assumed that there is a fourth aspect, a fourth sound of 'OM', which is simply referred to as 'the Fourth'. This is the inaudible dimension of 'OM'. Thus, 'OM' consists of four parts 'A', 'U', 'M' and 'the Fourth'. In the following, the four parts of 'OM' will be explained.

'A' is the first sound. 'A' is the beginning of the alphabet, not only in India but also in Western cultures. When we wake up in the morning and stretch our bodies the first sound we often utter is the sound of 'A'. This is the case because the sound 'A' as the initial sound is produced in the back of the throat. 'A' is the first sound and as such a symbol of opening and of beginning. 'A' also represents everything which begins within human beings and in the world, and also stages in life when something new emerges. 'A' is also a form of consciousness, which is only possible when there is awareness – the state of being awake.

As was shown 'O' consists of the two sounds 'A' and 'U'. Consequently, the second sound of 'OM' is 'U'. 'U' is the sound of the middle. The sound of 'U' is produced between the sound of 'A', which is articulated in the back of the throat, and the final closing sounds, which are produced in the front of the mouth with the lips. Thus, 'U' can be seen as a symbol of 'being in between', of going through change or of being on the path. 'U' represents stages in life of transition. As a form of consciousness 'U' represents the state in between being awake and deep sleep – the dream state.

The third and final sound is 'M'. 'M' is produced in the front of the mouth with the lips, but only if these are closed. Consequently, if the production of sound starts in the back of the throat with the opening of 'A' it ends in the front of the mouth with the lips and the closing sound 'M'. Hence, 'M' is the symbol of closure, of return, of homecoming and arriving, of retreat. In a positive sense, it is the end of a stage in life, but also one of destruction in a negative sense. As a form of consciousness 'M' means deep sleep and the end of any activities of consciousness.

Accordingly, 'A', 'U' and 'M' can be seen as representatives of all sounds one can produce. They are the symbols of all beginnings, of everything in between and of everything that will come to an end. They express any possible stages in the life of a human being and at the same time all conceivable conditions in the world. As such 'OM' is considered to be the symbol of the entire universe. As the representation of the three states of consciousness 'OM' covers all of them: being awake, the dream state and deep sleep. But 'OM' is even more. This 'more' is the fourth part of 'OM' and it is crucial.

The big question remains, what is meant by this fourth inaudible part of 'OM'. What more can there be that can be expressed through sound? What reaches beyond the beginning, the stages in between and the end? What fourth form of consciousness can one experience, which lay beyond being awake, dreaming or deep sleep? This is a dimension of 'OM', which can neither be expressed through audible sound nor through words. Hence, when the old texts refer to 'the Fourth' they more often use negations to describe it. 'The Fourth' is neither recognizable, nor tangible, nor perceptible and it cannot be described either. It is not even possible to find an appropriate term for it, thus it is only formally referred to as 'the Fourth'. And yet, this 'Fourth' that is described here so plainly and unimposingly is about the essence of the true Self, the experience of divine repose in the true Self, an awakening for inner bliss, which cannot be accomplished externally.

When man is in the state of everyday consciousness he can only perceive the audible sounds of 'OM' as the everyday consciousness only knows the apparent universe. Even with the highest effort it is not possible to go beyond waking, dreaming and deep sleep. This is so because the experience of 'the Fourth' cannot be achieved with effort. The inaudible fourth sound of OM can only be experienced through 'doing less', which is so much more than anything man can ever achieve. Practicing with the *mantra* 'OM' has got the potential to encourage this 'doing less'. Through continuous and permanent repetition of the *mantra* 'OM' in recitation or meditation, one's concentration can become more subtle. Serenity and inner calmness begin to increase. Attachments, addictions, urges and the unawareness of everyday consciousness begin to dissolve. In this yogic process psyche and mind become permeable and more transparent for a fundamental root dimension of reality. It becomes feasible that the fourth part of 'OM', the consciousness of the true Self, awakens, which reaches beyond being awake, dreaming or deep sleep. Regardless of where one lives, whether one is at the beginning of an action, in the middle or has just reached the end of it, one is always borne by this fundamental, divine force. This force has been given many names in the history of yoga and yet it cannot be grasped through any terminology. Only through letting go of the tangible sounds the experience of being borne can be experienced – the experience of 'the Fourth' as the resolution of the philosophy of 'OM'.

Exercise

The following exercise consists of three parts.

1. The experience of chanting the sounds 'A', 'U' and 'M':

- *Withdraw to a space where you can chant peacefully. Perhaps start with the sound of 'U' or 'I' and then try to move the production of the sounds further towards the back of the throat until you can essentially feel that 'A' is produced furthest in the back of the throat and thus is the initial sound man can produce.*
- *Next, chant the sounds 'O' and 'U' and feel where these sounds are produced. Try to explore that 'O' is produced right in the middle of 'A' and 'U' and thus is the confluence of 'A' and 'U'.*
- *Now, move further to the front of the mouth and experience the production of the closing sound 'M' by closing the lips.*
- *Finally, chant the sounds of 'A', 'U' and 'M' a couple of times and focus on the location of the sound production in the mouth. Feel: how 'A' is produced in the back of the throat as the opening sound, how 'U' is produced in the middle of the mouth and how the 'M' closes the chant in the front of the mouth.*

2. The symbolism of 'A', 'U' and 'M':

- *In your life are you in an 'A'-phase at the moment? Are you in the beginning of something or is the beginning of something dominating your life? Is something new emerging?*
- *Or is it more likely that you are in a 'U'-phase? Are you somewhere in between something, in a phase of transition or change or are you on the pathway of something?*
- *Or is 'M' dominating your life at the moment? Are you at the end of something, perhaps in the sense of returning or arriving, or in the sense of completion or even destruction?*
- *Can you give distinct answers to these questions or is there an*

overlap of various phases happening in your life?

Bring to mind how in your life you can go through an 'A'-, 'U'- or 'M'-phase and how at the same time these stages are ever changing. When reciting the mantra 'OM' over a period of time, one 'OM' is proceeded by another. Likewise, the beginning is followed by something in between until this comes to an end and a new beginning emerges: All our efforts, our life and our actions are determined by this repetitious process of beginning, being in between and finalizing in order to advance forward.

3. The experience of 'the Fourth':

Again chant the mantra 'OM', preferably in a circle or in a group.

- *First, focus on the action of deliberately producing and creating the sound of 'OM'. Hence, the focus is on the tangible, audible part of 'OM'.*
- *'The Fourth' can emerge when you begin to do less and also when you do not exert yourself. With less effort a certain force of the chanting can emerge. Let your chanting be carried by the dynamic of the group, or if you are practicing by yourself feel the vibrations of the space.*

When you practice this exercise with endurance and over a long period of time, it is very likely that you will experience 'more' by doing less and that you will benefit from a power, force or energy, which is not 'done' by yourself and which cannot be realized through 'doing'. Then it becomes feasible that 'OM' will unfold to the full potential of all four parts.

18

Divine and Self-Experience

In the various religions there are many differing concepts of god. Often god is considered a being somewhere beyond. God is in heaven, whereas man remains on earth. It is one of the great discoveries of yoga that god is much closer to man than was generally believed. Yoga is the pathway of training the consciousness in order to be able to see what man really is. According to yoga, the true Self of man, which is referred to as *atman* in Sanskrit, is one with *brahman*, 'the Absolute'. The old *Upanishads* state the following on this divine experience as the experience of the true Self:

> *Then the words merge with the mind and yet they do not grasp it.*
> *(Taittiriya Upanishad 2.9)*

'Absolute' and 'Self', *brahman* and *atman*, are terms for something which cannot be grasped with any words. They are terms for the experience of the unspeakable and the unthinkable. Yet, it was tried again and again to call this unspeakable and unthinkable by a name. Even this chapter on divine and Self-experience is yet another attempt to explain this ineffable experience from where all words reverse without grasping it. It is another attempt to contemplate this experience philosophically, again through the use of many words.

Each time we speak, write or read we inevitably have to make use of words that spring from the mind, but now we are trying to aim at something which is to be found further inside than can be grasped by mind. Consequently, it is important to go beyond the words and look towards the experience, to which the words can only point. A common method to do so is through the use of negations as was done by the great sage *Yajnavalkya* in the *Upanishads*. When *Yajnavalkya* referred to the experience of *brahman* he said:

Neti neti – It is neither this nor this.
(Brihadaranyaka Upanishad 4.5.15)

It is indeed possible to purposefully describe the material world. Likewise, we can analyze the processes of our lives through the use of thoughts. Logic is also tangible. *Brahman*, however, is to be found in a deeper place, beyond any thought. Initially, we can use words to approach *brahman*, but at a certain point we have to let go of them as if we were jumping off a cliff and thus negate all words for *brahman*: It is neither called this nor that.

Ramakrishna, a great Indian sage from the 19th century, described that pathway to the experience of *brahman* in the following beautiful image:

A doll made of salt wanted to explore the depth of the ocean. It wanted to tell others how deep the ocean is. But how could it? As soon as it touched the ocean, the doll dissolved. Who now could tell the others about the depth of the ocean?
(Sri Ramakrishna)

Our thoughts are like this doll that wanted to explore the depth of the ocean. Of course, it is possible to develop comprehensive theories in order to understand *brahman* through cognition. Yet, all theories remain strange as long as we look at them from the outside and analytically. If one has not entered the path of yoga yet, he can only speculate about the deeper meaning of yoga and what is meant by divine experience such as the experience of *brahman*. It is crucial, however, to let oneself in for the experience and walk into the ocean like the salt doll does. But what happens once the doll touches the ocean? The doll dissolves and becomes one with the ocean. The same will happen when we let our cognitive self in for the experience of *brahman*. Thoughts about god will dissolve once the practitioner will break through to the experience of yoga. Instead of contemplating 'the Absolute' the practitioner will recognize himself as *brahman*. Accordingly, the *Upanishads* state:

> He who knows the supreme brahman becomes brahman.
> (Mundaka Upanishad 3.2.9)

In order to essentially get to know *brahman*, one has to let go of all concepts of what the experience of *brahman* could be. The one who knows *brahman* lives from it and is one with it without the need to even utter a single word about it. When the salt doll dissolves into the ocean not only do all words and thoughts dissolve, but also all tensions, all ties, attachments and unconsciousness and with it we ourselves dissolve. Consequently, the salt doll is an image of our Self. Accordingly, *Yajnavalkya* says:

> 'Not' can be seen only after death
> (Brihadaranyaka Upanishad 2.4.12)

When referring to 'death' *Yajnavalkya* does not mean the physical death of the body at the end of our earthly lives, but what he refers to is the union with *brahman*. Our human body can be compared to an old snakeskin that has been shed on an anthill. In this image from the *Upanishads* the snakeskin is dead and yet it moves. The skin's movement, however, does not come from itself, but because it is carried by ants.

This image shows that the union of man and *brahman* is not so much an experience of looking up to a god. Neither is it about an inflated ego, which has become as big as a god. Rather, being on the yogic pathway means a 'doing less', or 'doing nothing' and finally it means 'dying'. But who is dying? The ego is dying, which is our apparent 'I' of attachments and unconsciousness. Consequently, being on the yogic pathway means to be on a path of inner poise. It is the letting go of self-centeredness but also of heteronomy, of ties, attachments or compulsions, which usually define the 'I' of everyday consciousness.

Just like a dead snakeskin shed on an anthill does not move by itself, but is carried by ants, so man is carried by the experience of a divine life. Hence, yoga is the discovery of a divine life, which springs from this very depth of the true Self. A divine life does not materialize from the outside, but it arises from the essence of one's own existence. Through the experience of *brahman*, 'the Absolute', man can return home, to his true Self, to *atman*. From the perspective of yoga, divine experience means to awaken to one's true Self.

Divine and Self-Experience

Exercise

The Upanishads name two images, which can help us to understand yoga as a pathway of divine experience. The first image is that of a salt doll dissolving in the ocean. The second image is the one of a dead snakeskin shed on an anthill. Now bring to mind your own yoga practice and ask yourself the following questions:

- *In your yoga practice have you ever experienced that you do not need to exert yourself so much anymore and hence you do less?*
- *Reflect how through 'doing less' your 'I-ness' may begin to dissolve like the salt doll in an ocean. Can you describe such an experience?*
- *Have you ever experienced being carried by a new kind of energy when you let go and do less, just like a dead snakeskin is moved by ants as in the second image of the Upanishads?*
- *How would you describe this kind of new energy?*

Now you have reached a point in your yogic experience where words and thoughts may begin to reverse without quite grasping it. It is important that in today's world we can find our own language that will point towards the inner treasure of yoga, independent of whether we choose religious language or any other means of expression that we consider more appropriate.

MANTRA BOOKS

We publish books on Eastern religions and philosophies.
Books that aim to inform and explore the various
traditions, that began rooted in East and
have migrated West.